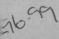
Video 8.2   **Non-Surgical Body Contouring: Cellulite**

Thomas E. Rohrer, MD

Video 9   **Thermage Monopolar Radiofrequency**

Michael S. Kaminer, MD

Melissa Bogle, MD

Video 10   **Laser Treatment of Ethnic Skin**

Stephanie G.Y. Ho, MD

Henry H.L. Chan, MD

ALREADY REGISTERED?
1. Log in at expertconsult.com
2. Scratch off your Activation Code below
3. Enter it into the "Add a Title" box
4. Click "Activate Now"
5. Click the title under "My Titles"

FIRST-TIME USER?
1. *REGISTER*
- Click "Register Now" at expertconsult.com
- Fill in your user information and click "Continue"
2. *ACTIVATE YOUR BOOK*
- Scratch off your Activation Code below
- Enter it into the "Enter Activation Code" box
- Click "Activate Now"
- Click the title under "My Titles"

Lasers and Lights

Procedures in Cosmetic Dermatology
Series Editor; Jeffrey S. Dover MD, FRCPC, FRCP
Associate Editor: Murad Alam MD

Chemical Peels
Second edition
Rebecca C. Tung, MD and Mark G. Rubin MD
ISBN 978-1-4377-1924-6

Treatment of Leg Veins
Second edition
Murad Alam, MD and Sirunya Silapunt, MD
ISBN 978-1-4377-0739-7

Body Contouring
Bruse E Katz MD and Neil S Sadick MD FAAD FAACS
FACP FACPh
ISBN 978-1-4377-0739-7

Non Surgical Skin Tightening and Lifting
Murad Alam MD MSCI
and Jeffrey S Dover MD RCPC FRCP
ISBN 978-1-4160-5960-8

Botulinum Toxin
Third Edition
Alastair Carruthers MA BM BCh FRCPC FRCP(Lon) and
Jean Carruthers MD FRCSC FRC(Ophth) FASOPRS
ISBN 978-1-4557-2781-0

Soft Tissue Augmentation
Third Edition
Jean Carruthers MD FRCSC FRC(Ophth) FASOPRS and
Alastair Carruthers MA BM BCh FRCPC FRCP(Lon)
ISBN 978-1-4557-2782-7

Cosmeceuticals
Second edition
Zoe-Diana Draelos MD
ISBN 978-1-4160-5553-2

Lasers and Lights
Third edition
George Hruza MD and Mathew Avram MD
ISBN 978-1-4557-2783-4

Photodynamic Therapy
Second edition
Mitchel P. Goldman MD
ISBN 978-1-4160-4211-2

Liposuction
C. William Hanke MD MPH FACP and Gerhard Sattler MD
ISBN 978-1-4160-2208-4

Scar Revision
Kenneth A Arndt MD
ISBN 978-1-4160-3131-4

Hair Transplantation
Robert S. Haber MD and Dowling B Stough MD
ISBN 978-1-4160-3104-8

Blepharoplasty
Ronald L. Moy MD and Edgar F Fincher MD
ISBN 978-1-4160-2996-0

Advanced Face Lifting
Ronald L. Moy MD and Edgar F Fincher MD
ISBN 978-1-4160-2997-7

For Elsevier

Content Strategist: Belinda Kuhn
Content Development Specialist: Martin Mellor Publishing Services Ltd
Project Manager: Sruthi Viswam
Design: Miles Hitchen
Illustration Manager: Jennifer Rose
Marketing Manager: Carla Holloway

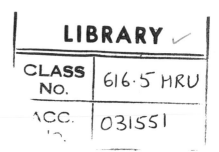

3rd Edition

PROCEDURES IN COSMETIC DERMATOLOGY

Lasers and Lights

Edited by

George J. Hruza MD, MBA
Clinical Professor, Dermatology, Saint Louis University, Saint Louis;
Medical Director, Laser & Dermatologic Surgery Center, Chesterfield, MO, USA

Mathew M. Avram MD, JD
Assistant Professor of Dermatology, Harvard Medical School;
Affiliate Faculty, Wellman Centerfor Photomedicine;
Director, Massachusetts General Hospital Dermatology Laser & Cosmetic Center, Boston, MA, USA

Series Editor
Jeffrey S. Dover MD, FRCPC, FRCP
Associate Professor of Clinical Dermatology, Yale University School of Medicine, New Haven, CT;
Adjunct Professor of Medicine (Dermatology), Dartmouth Medical School, Hanover, NH;
Adjunct Associate Professor of Dermatology, Brown Medical School, Providence, RI;
Director, SkinCare Physicians, Chestnut Hill, MA, USA

Associate Editor
Murad Alam MD
Professor of Dermatology, Otolaryngology, and Surgery;
Chief, Section of Cutaneous and Aesthetic Surgery,
Northwestern University, Chicago, IL, USA

Expert CONSULT
For additional online content visit expertconsult.com

SAUNDERS

ELSEVIER

London New York Oxford St Louis Sydney Toronto 2013

ELSEVIER
SAUNDERS

SAUNDERS is an imprint of Elsevier Inc.

First edition 2005
Second edition 2009
Third edition 2013

Notices

Knowledge and best practice in this field are constantly changing. As new research and experience broaden our understanding, changes in research methods, professional practices, or medical treatment may become necessary.

Practitioners and researchers must always rely on their own experience and knowledge in evaluating and using any information, methods, compounds, or experiments described herein. In using such information or methods they should be mindful of their own safety and the safety of others, including parties for whom they have a professional responsibility.

With respect to any drug or pharmaceutical products identified, readers are advised to check the most current information provided (i) on procedures featured or (ii) by the manufacturer of each product to be administered, to verify the recommended dose or formula, the method and duration of administration, and contraindications. It is the responsibility of practitioners, relying on their own experience and knowledge of their patients, to make diagnoses, to determine dosages and the best treatment for each individual patient, and to take all appropriate safety precautions.

To the fullest extent of the law, neither the Publisher nor the authors, contributors, or editors, assume any liability for any injury and/or damage to persons or property as a matter of products liability, negligence or otherwise, or from any use or operation of any methods, products, instructions, or ideas contained in the material herein.

ISBN: 978-1-4557-2783-4
Ebook ISBN: 978-1-4557-3778-9

Printed in China

Last digit is the print number: 9 8 7 6 5 4 3 2 1

Seven years ago we embarked on an effort to produce *Procedures in Cosmetic Dermatology*, a series of high quality, practical, up-to-date, illustrated manuals. Our plan was to provide dermatologists, dermatologic surgeons, and others dedicated to the pursuit of functional knowledge with detailed portable books accompanied by high quality "how to" DVD's containing all the information they needed to master most, if not all, of the leading edge cosmetic techniques. Thanks to the efforts of world class volume editors, master chapter authors, and the tireless and extraordinary publishing staff at Elsevier, the series has been more successful than any of us could have imagined. Over the past seven years, 15 distinct volumes have been introduced, and have been purchased by thousands of physicians all over the world. Originally published in English, many of the texts have been translated into different languages including Italian, French, Spanish, Chinese, Polish, Korean, Portuguese, and Russian.

Our commitment has always been to ensure that the practical, easy to use information conveyed in the series is also extremely up-to-date, incorporating all the latest methods and materials. To that end, given the rapidly changing nature of our subspecialty, the time has now come to inaugurate the third edition. During the next few years, refined, enlarged, and improved texts will be released in a sequential manner. The most time-sensitive books will be revised first, and others will follow.

This series is an ever evolving project. So in addition to third editions of current books, we will be introducing entirely new books to cover novel procedures that may not have existed when the series began. Enjoy and keep learning.

Jeffrey S. Dover MD FRCPC and
Murad Alam MD, MSCI

While dermatologists have been procedurally inclined since the beginning of the specialty, particularly rapid change has occurred in the past quarter century. The advent of frozen section technique and the golden age of Mohs skin cancer surgery has led to the formal incorporation of surgery within the dermatology curriculum. More recently technological breakthroughs in minimally invasive procedural dermatology have offered an aging population new options for improving the appearance of damaged skin.

Procedures for rejuvenating the skin and adjacent regions are actively sought by our patients. Significantly, dermatologists have pioneered devices, technologies and medications, which have continued to evolve at a startling pace. Numerous major advances, including virtually all cutaneous lasers and light-source-based procedures, botulinum exotoxin, soft tissue augmentation, dilute anesthesia liposuction, leg vein treatments, chemical peels, and hair transplants have been invented, or developed and enhanced by dermatologists. Dermatologists understand procedures and we have special insight into the structure, function, and working of skin. Cosmetic dermatologists have made rejuvenation accessible to risk-averse patients by emphasizing safety and reducing operative trauma. No specialty is better positioned than dermatology to lead the field of cutaneous surgery while meeting patient needs.

As dermatology grows as a specialty, an ever-increasing proportion of dermatologists will become proficient in the delivery of different procedures. Not all dermatologists will perform all procedures, and some will perform very few, but even the less procedurally directed amongst us must be well-versed in the details to be able to guide and educate our patients. Whether you are a skilled dermatologic surgeon interested in further expanding your surgical repertoire, a complete surgical novice wishing to learn a few simple procedures, or somewhere in between, this book and this series are for you.

The volume you are holding is one of a series entitled *Procedures in Cosmetic Dermatology*. The purpose of each book is to serve as a practical primer on a major topic area in procedural dermatology.

If you want to make sure you find the right book for your needs, you may wish to know what this book is and what it is not. It is not a comprehensive text grounded in theoretical underpinnings. It is not exhaustively referenced. It is not designed to be a completely unbiased review of the world's literature on the subject. At the same time, it is not an overview of cosmetic procedures that describes these in generalities without providing enough specific information to actually permit someone to perform the procedures. And importantly, it is not so heavy that it can serve as a doorstop or a shelf filler.

What this book and this series offer is a step-by-step, practical guide to performing cutaneous surgical procedures. Each volume in the series has been edited by a known authority in that subfield. Each editor has recruited other equally practical-minded, technically skilled, hands-on clinicians to write the constituent chapters. Most chapters have two authors to ensure that different approaches and a broad range of opinions are incorporated. On the other hand, the two authors and the editors also collectively provide a consistency of tone. A uniform template has been used within each chapter so that the reader will be easily able to navigate all the books in the series. Within every chapter, the authors succinctly tell it like they do it. The emphasis is on therapeutic technique; treatment methods are discussed with an eye to appropriate indications, adverse events, and unusual cases. Finally, this book is short and can be read in its entirety on a long plane ride. We believe that brevity paradoxically results in greater information transfer because cover-to-cover mastery is practicable.

We hope you enjoy this book and the rest of the books in the series and that you benefit from the many hours of clinical wisdom that have been distilled to produce it. Please keep it nearby, where you can reach for it when you need it.

Jeffrey S. Dover MD FRCPC and Murad Alam MD

This third edition of *Lasers and Lights* thoroughly details the manifold developments within our field since the last edition by some of the leaders in the field of laser surgery. New techniques are emphasized in the updated video clips that accompany this edition. The organization of chapter topics reflects these changes. In fact, there are a few entire chapters on treatments that did not exist at the time of the prior edition, and the rest of the chapters have been completely rewritten and updated. The book starts with an excellent overview of the basic science behind these devices written by Rox Anderson and his colleagues that provides a comprehensive overview of this field. The subsequent chapter topics include: treatment of cutaneous vascular lesions, laser hair removal, nonablative laser and light skin rejuvenation, nonablative fractional resurfacing, ablative fractional resurfacing, laser resurfacing, non-surgical body contouring, non-surgical tissue tightening,

laser treatment of ethnic skin, and complications and legal considerations of laser and light treatments. These chapters are written for the benefit of novice as well as experienced laser surgeons with an eye towards practical, yet comprehensive, overviews of these diverse topics. Patient selection, treatment strategies, laser safety are all emphasized throughout the text. Basic and advanced techniques are explained in a straightforward manner. Extensive photographic and graphic illustration, practical pearls, tables, clinical cases, key points and charts are an invaluable addition to the written text. In sum, *Lasers and Lights* provides an outstanding overview of the use of laser and light sources within the field of cosmetic dermatology.

George J. Hruza and Mathew M. Avram
August 2012

R. Rox Anderson MD
Professor of Dermatology, Harvard Medical School; Director, Wellman Center for Photomedicine, Department of Dermatology, Massachusetts General Hospital, Harvard Medical School, Boston, MA, USA

Lawrence S. Bass MD, FACS
Director, Minimally Invasive Plastic Surgery; Clinical Assistant Professor of Plastic Surgery, Department of Plastic Surgery, NYU School of Medicine, New York, NY, USA

Travis W. Blalock MD
Procedural Dermatology Fellow, Division of Dermatology and Dermatologic Surgery, Scripps Clinic, La Jolla, CA, USA

Melissa A. Bogle MD
Director, The Laser and Cosmetic Surgery Center of Houston; Associate Clinical Professor, The University of Texas Anderson Cancer Center, Houston, TX, USA

Chung-Yin Stanley Chan MD
Procedural Dermatology Fellow, SkinCare Physicians, Chestnut Hill, MA, USA

Henry H.L. Chan MD, PhD, MBBS, MSc, MRCP, FRCP, FHKCP, FHKAM
Honorary Clinical Professor, Division of Dermatology, Department of Medicine, University of Hong Kong; Honorary Consultant Dermatologist, Queen Mary Hospital, Hong Kong, China; Visiting Scientist, Wellman Center for Photomedicine, Massachusetts General Hospital, Harvard Medical School, Boston, MA, USA

Barry E. DiBernardo MD, FACS
Director, New Jersey Plastic Surgery, Montclair, NJ; Clinical Associate Professor, Department of Surgery, Division of Plastic Surgery, University of Medicine and Dentistry of New Jersey, Newark, NJ, USA

Jeffrey S. Dover MD, FRCPC, FRCP
Associate Professor of Clinical Dermatology, Yale University School of Medicine, New Haven, CT; Adjunct Professor of Medicine (Dermatology), Dartmouth Medical School, Hanover, NH; Adjunct Associate Professor of Dermatology, Brown Medical School, Providence, RI; Director, SkinCare Physicians, Chestnut Hill, MA, USA

David J. Goldberg MD, JD
Director, Skin Laser and Surgery Specialists of New York and New Jersey, Hackensack, NJ; Clinical Professor of Dermatology and Director of Laser Research, Mount Sinai Medical School, New York, NY; Clinical Professor of Dermatology and Director of Dermatologic Surgery, UMDNJ-New Jersey Medical School, NJ; Adjunct Professor of Law, Fordham Law School, New York, NY, USA

Stephanie G.Y. Ho MB CHB, MRCP
Clinical Associate, Department of Medicine, Division of Dermatology, University of Hong Kong, Hong Kong, China

Omar A. Ibrahimi MD, PhD
Assistant Professor of Dermatology, Dermatologic & Mohs Surgery; Director, Cutaneous Laser and Cosmetic Surgery, Department of Dermatology, University of Connecticut Health Center, Farmington, CT; Visiting Assistant Professor of Dermatology, Wellman Center for Photomedicine, Massachusetts General Hospital, Harvard Medical School, Cambridge, MA, USA

H. Ray Jalian MD
Clinical Research Fellow, Wellman Center for Photomedicine, Department of Dermatology, Massachusetts General Hospital, Harvard Medical School, Boston, MA, USA

Michael S. Kaminer MD
Assistant Professor of Clinical Dermatology, Yale University School of Medicine, New Haven, CT; Adjunct Assistant Professor of Medicine (Dermatology), Dartmouth Medical School, Hanover, NH; Adjunct Assistant Professor of Dermatology, Brown Medical School; Managing Partner, SkinCare Physicians, Chestnut Hill, MA, USA

Kristen M. Kelly MD
Associate Professor, Dermatology and Surgery, University of California, Irvine, CA, USA

Suzanne L. Kilmer MD
Director, Laser and Skin Surgery Center of Northern California, Sacramento; Associate Clinical Professor, Department of Dermatology, University of CA, Davis School of Medicine, CA, USA

Jeremy Man MD, FRCPC
Physician at Skin Laser and Surgery Specialists of New York, NY and New Jersey, NJ, USA

Kavita Mariwalla MD
Assistant Clinical Professor, Department of Dermatology, Columbia University, New York, NY, USA

Andrei Metelitsa MD, FRCPC, FAAD
Clinical Assistant Professor, Division of Dermatology, University of Calgary; Co-Director, Institute for Skin Advancement, Calgary, AB, Canada

Andrew A. Nelson MD
Private Practice, Nelson Dermatology, St. Petersburg, FL; Assistant Clinical Professor, Department of Dermatology, Tufts University School of Medicine, Boston, MA, USA

Jason N. Pozner MD, FACS
Director; Co-Owner, Sanctuary Plastic Surgery; Affiliate Assistant Professor of Clinical Biomedical Science, Charles E. Schmidt College of Medicine, Florida Atlantic University, Boca Raton; Adjunct Clinical Faculty, Department of Plastic Surgery, Cleveland Clinic, Weston, FL, USA

E. Victor Ross MD
Director, Cosmetic and Laser Dermatology Unit, Scripps
Clinic, San Diego, CA, USA

Iris Kedar Rubin MD
Consultant, Children's National Medical Center, Washington
DC; Dermatology Center, Bethesda, MD, USA

Fernanda H. Sakamoto MD, PhD
Instructor in Dermatology, Harvard Medical School; Assistant
in Research, Wellman Center for Photomedicine, Department
of Dermatology, Massachusetts General Hospital, Boston,
MA, USA

To my Hrilliams family: my wife Carrie Hruza and our children, Stephanie and Paul Hruza and Hope and Rose Williams for giving my life joy and fulfillment. And to my parents Drs. Judita and Zdenek Hruza for their unwavering support and love

George J. Hruza

To Alison, whose grace, beauty, love and support inspire me each day.

To Rachel, Alexander and Noah who are my heart and soul.

To my parents, Morrell and Maria Avram, for their unconditional love from the day I was born.

Mathew Avram

To the women in my life: my grandmothers, Bertha and Lillian, my mother, Nina, my daughters, Sophie and Isabel, and especially to my wife, Tania. For their never-ending encouragement, patience, support, love, and friendship

To my father, Mark – a great teacher and role model

To my mentor, Kenneth A. Arndt for his generosity, kindness, sense of humor, joie de vivre, and above all else curiosity and enthusiasm

Jeffrey S. Dover

Elsevier's dedicated editorial staff has made possible the continuing success of this ambitious project. The new team led by Belinda Kuhn, Martin Mellor and the production staff have refined the concept for the second edition while maintaining the series' reputation for quality and cutting-edge relevance. In this, they have been ably supported by the graphics shop, which has created the signature high quality illustrations and layouts that are the backbone of each book. We are also deeply grateful to the volume editors, who have generously found time in their schedules, cheerfully accepted our guidelines, and recruited the most knowledgeable chapter authors. And we especially thank the chapter contributors, without whose work there would be no books at all. Finally, I would also like to convey my debt to my teachers, Kenneth Arndt, Jeffrey Dover, Michael Kaminer, Leonard Goldberg, and David Bickers, and my parents, Rahat and Rehana Alam.

Murad Alam

Understanding lasers, lights, and tissue interactions

Fernanda H. Sakamoto, H. Ray Jalian, R. Rox Anderson

1

Summary and Key Features

- Lasers and flashlamps can destroy histological targets using the concept of selective photothermolysis (SP)

- Ablative lasers vaporize tissue; non-ablative lasers heat tissue without vaporization

- Selective histological damage requires heat confinement to desirable target structures. Selective photothermolysis combines appropriate wavelength ('color' of light), fluence ('dose' of light), pulse duration, and protective skin cooling for the treatment of a variety of diseases

- Understanding the optical and thermal properties of skin and its histological targets allows safe and optimal treatments using light sources

Light

Light is a fundamental form of energy with numerous medical applications. At the quantum level, light is composed of packets of energy, known as photons. Each photon carries a discrete amount of energy. Light is also an electromagnetic wave. The electromagnetic spectrum extends from low frequency radio waves to ultra-high-energy gamma rays. The energy carried by each photon is determined by its wavelength, which for visible light (400–700 nm) corresponds to its color. Laser is an acronym for *light amplification by the stimulated emission of radiation*. Stimulated emission is a quantum process by which one photon can stimulate the creation of another photon, by interacting with an excited atom or molecule. Lasers work by pumping many atoms into the excited state, from which a very large amount of stimulated emission can occur. Laser light is typically monochromatic, meaning that the output is composed of a single wavelength of light. A second characteristic of lasers is coherence, meaning that all waves of light travel in phase spatially and temporally. Laser light is also highly collimated, which allows the laser beam to travel long distances without divergence, and to be focused to a spot about equal to its own wavelength. These properties of lasers allow for unique forms of in vivo imaging, such as confocal microscopy and optical coherence tomography.

Lasers are also capable of producing extremely intense, short pulses of light. In dermatology and ophthalmology, pulsed lasers have become mainstream tools for precise surgery and target-selective treatments. Prior to 1983, lasers in dermatology were used primarily for non-specific tissue destruction. With the description of the theory of **selective photothermolysis** (SP) by Anderson & Parrish in 1983, applications of lasers in dermatology have evolved to a host of devices for more precise, targeted thermal damage, while minimizing non-specific tissue destruction. Non-laser flashlamp sources called intense pulsed light (IPL) have also been developed for some of the applications of SP that use millisecond pulses of light. Understanding the theory of SP is vital for making sense of the large number of laser and IPL devices and applications. An understanding of the optical properties of skin is also needed, since the whole endeavor of laser treatment starts with the absorption of light energy, inside the skin.

Lasers that vaporize a thin layer or column of tissue have also been developed. The concept of **fractional photothermolysis** (FP), reported by Manstein and colleagues in 2004, recently launched another era of lasers in dermatology, in which patterns of very small non-selective thermal damage zones are used to stimulate skin remodeling without scarring. Laser-stimulated remodeling is a complex process that mimics large wound healing in some aspects, with epidermal regeneration, induction of metalloproteinases, and formation of new dermal matrix including elastin fibrils and collagen types I and III. Compared with gross wound healing, there is minimal inflammation and no scarring. A 'cookbook' approach should be avoided when choosing among these devices for various applications. When treating a particular patient with a particular device, a combination of fundamental understanding, careful observation of the appropriate clinical end points, dexterity, and clinical experience is far better than a set of instructions (Box 1.1).

Light interactions with skin

Photons can be **absorbed** (giving up their energy to matter) or **scattered** (changing their direction of travel). Light that is scattered back from skin is called reflectance. For a given skin layer, light that passes through it is called transmittance. Scattering is inversely wavelength dependent, such that shorter wavelengths are scattered more and longer wavelengths (such as infrared) are scattered less. We are all familiar with these events – black objects become hot when placed in sunlight due to absorption and water droplets (clouds) or crystals (snow) appear bright white because they strongly scatter light, with little or no absorption. Similarly, light is both absorbed and scattered within the skin. Thus, skin layers are cloudy and colored depending on the mix of scattering and absorption. Penetration of light into (and beyond) skin is limited by both absorption and scattering. All effects of light on the skin begin with photon absorption, and the molecules that absorb light are called **chromophores**. Ablative lasers are those that vaporize tissue by rapidly boiling water inside the tissue. It should come as no surprise therefore, that the lasers intended for skin ablation are at wavelengths strongly absorbed by water. Non-ablative lasers do not vaporize tissue. There are many non-ablative lasers in dermatology, some of which are at wavelengths absorbed by water and some of which are absorbed by other chromophores such as melanin and/or hemoglobins.

Pearl 1

Ablative light sources vaporize the skin while non-ablative and selective laser treatments can be performed only with selective photothermolysis.

Laser dosimetry is extremely important for safe and effective results. In order to remove tissue, ablative lasers must raise local tissue temperature beyond the boiling point of 100°C, plus add much more energy needed for changing water into steam. The fundamental unit of **energy** is a joule (J). It takes 4.2 J to heat 1 cm^3 of water by 1°C. In order to vaporize the same 1 cm^3 of water, more than 2000 J are required. An ablative laser must deliver about 2500 J of energy per cm^3 of vaporized tissue. Not only is a lot of energy required to ablate skin tissue – the energy must be delivered quickly to remove the hot tissue before heat is conducted deeply into the skin, causing a burn. The standard ablative lasers in dermatology are erbium (2940 nm) and CO_2 (10 600 nm). The desired interaction of these ablative lasers is to precisely remove a thin layer for resurfacing or narrow column for fractional treatment of skin, leaving behind minimal residual thermal damage. A thin residual thermal damage layer, typically about 0.1 mm, is useful in practice for hemostasis. Minimum residual thermal injury is achieved with ablative lasers by a combination of wavelength, pulse duration, and power density (W/cm^2) at the skin surface. A common mistake made by beginning laser users is to 'turn down' the power of a surgical CO_2 laser in a misguided attempt to exercise caution. Unfortunately, turning down the power can cause burns because the process turns from rapid, precise vaporization with minimal thermal damage to bulk heating of the skin from unwanted residual heat. Fortunately, many of the ablative lasers made specifically for dermatology are designed to stay within a range of dosimetry for rapid tissue ablation, making this scenario less likely. The safest erbium and CO_2 lasers are those emitting high power, high energy, and short (less than a few ms) pulses, designed specifically for dermatologic use with minimal residual thermal damage. Despite whatever safeguards an ablative laser may offer, the most reliable safeguard is an ability to recognize the desired and undesired immediate response end points. For example, immediate contraction of the skin is always a sign that substantial thermal injury of the dermis has occurred (Fig. 1.1).

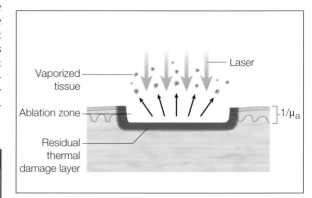

Figure 1.1 Scheme of ablative laser vaporizing skin, leaving a residual thermal damage layer.

Fluence is defined as the energy delivered per unit area of skin, and its units are typically expressed in J/cm^2. One can think of fluence as the local 'dose' of laser energy applied to skin. Pulse duration (also called pulsewidth, or exposure duration) is simply the time for which laser energy is delivered, expressed in seconds. Power is defined as the rate of energy delivery. Power is measured in watts (W), a familiar unit because of common devices such as light bulbs. One W is defined by 1 W = 1 J/second. A common incandescent light bulb consumes 100 W of electrical power, but emits less than 10 W of light. In contrast, common lasers in dermatology produce 10 to 1 000 000 000 (a billion) W of light power. The Q-switched lasers, which we commonly use to remove tattoos and pigmented lesions, produce more power than a typical nuclear power plant! However, these lasers emit that impressive power for only 10–100 nanoseconds (ns, billionths of a second). Thus, the fluence for treatment of a child with a nevus of Ota using a 10 ns Q-switched laser, and of a child with port-wine stain using a 1 millisecond (ms) pulsed dye laser, can be similar – about 5–10 J/cm^2 – but the pulsed dye laser has 100 000 times less power than the Q-switched laser.

Skin optics

In skin, the most important chromophores are hemoglobin, melanin, exogenous pigments (e.g. tattoo ink, some drugs), water, and lipids. The intended target chromophore, depth of the target structures, and absorption of light by adjacent tissue influence the appropriate wavelength selection. Absorption spectra of various chromophores across the electromagnetic spectrum are summarized in **Figure 1.2**.

Selective photothermolysis

SP relies on fundamental choices being made correctly – wavelength, pulse duration, fluence, exposure spot size,

and use of skin cooling. First, a wavelength (or, with IPLs, a range of wavelengths) must be used that is preferentially absorbed by the intended 'target' structures such as hair follicles, microvessels, tattoo inks, or melanocytes. Thus far, all lasers utilizing SP operate in the visible and near-infrared (NIR) spectrum. Generally, in the visible light spectrum, a target chromophore is treated using wavelengths of light of a complimentary color. For example, red tattoo ink absorbs green light and can be effectively treated with a frequency doubled Q-switched Nd:YAG laser operating at the green wavelength of 532 nm. Similarly, green tattoo ink is best removed with a red Q-switched laser, such as the ruby laser at 694 nm. Preferential absorption implies the avoidance of competing chromophores, not simply strong absorption in the intended target. For example, when treating dermal targets such as blood vessels it is important to minimize unwanted damage to the epidermis. Since every photon that reaches a blood vessel must first travel through the overlying epidermis, the best wavelengths for port-wine stain treatment are *not* simply those with strong absorption by blood. The proper wavelength(s) must also penetrate deeply enough to reach the intended targets. Across the visible and near-infrared spectrum from 400 to 1200 nm, longer wavelengths penetrate deeper into tissue. These reasons account for the use of yellow light pulsed dye lasers rather than the very strongly absorbed blue wavelengths for treating superficial vascular lesions. Long-pulsed dye lasers are the first example of a laser designed specifically for a medical application: treatment of port-wine stains in children (see Case study 2). On the microscopic scale, microvessels are selectively heated and damaged, with minimal injury to the rest of the skin structures. However, for a hypertrophic or deep vascular lesion, such as many adult port-wine stains and venous malformations, much better efficacy is often obtained using the deeply penetrating 755 nm near-infrared alexandrite laser, as detailed by Izikson et al in 2009. (Looking at **Fig. 1.2**, it is easy to observe that hemoglobin absorbs yellow light much more strongly than at 755 nm, a wavelength that is also well absorbed by melanin.) When alexandrite lasers are used for vascular lesion treatment, it is therefore imperative to use excellent skin cooling for epidermal protection; see Chang & Nelson 1999 and Altschuler et al 2000.

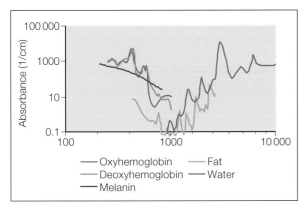

Figure 1.2 Absorption spectra of chromophores commonly used for selective photothermolysis laser surgery. *This figure was modified from Sakamoto et al, 2007.*

Pearl 2

Selective photothermolysis allows microscopic laser surgery of histological targets.

Pearl 3

Laser wavelength is usually the complementary color of the target chromophore (e.g. 'red' 694 nm Q-switched ruby laser to treat green tattoos).

Melanin absorbs across a wide spectrum of wavelengths. Eumelanin, the primary chromophore in the epidermis and darkly pigmented hair follicles, has a broad absorption spectrum spanning from ultraviolet light to the near-infrared region. Eumelanin is the chromophore targeted in lentigo simplex. It is also the target in laser hair removal with the secondary target being the follicular stem cells, as reported by Grossman and colleagues in 1996. In fair-skinned individuals with dark hair, wavelengths in the near-infrared range (810 nm diode; 755 nm alexandrite) are ideal for laser depilation. However, a common mistake is to use these popular devices for hair removal of red or blond hair, which is primarily composed of pheomelanin. These laser wavelengths are poorly absorbed by pheomelanin and are therefore ineffective for permanent removal of red or blond hair.

In general, water is not a useful target for selective photothermolyis because it is present at high concentration in almost every skin structure. Water absorption gradually increases starting in the near IR range and peaking within the mid-IR spectrum. When used in conjunction with appropriate epidermal cooling devices, lasers within this wavelength spectrum can function as non-ablative modalities for photorejuvenation by targeting water within the dermis, thereby generating heat and controlled thermal damage. This wounding of the dermis subsequently results in collagen remodeling, as well as neocollagenesis, contributing to the modest improvement in the appearance of rhytides.

More recently, near-infrared lasers have been used by Sakamoto and co-workers and by Anderson et al to target lipid-rich tissue. Unlike the targeting of traditional chromophores, which is based on electronic charge, lasers to target lipids are based on the vibrational modes of the molecules. Lipid molecules are selectively destroyed at 1210 nm and 1720 nm where their absorption is slightly higher than that of water. Although there are no commercial devices yet available, the application of these forthcoming devices offers an appealing, alternative, non-invasive methodology of targeting lipids.

The second essential factor for SP is to use a **pulse duration** that allows heat to be confined during the laser pulse in or near the target structures. The moment that heat is formed in a target by preferential absorption of photons, the target begins to cool by conduction. Therefore, heating of the target is a balance between the rate of photon absorption and the rate of cooling. The concept of a particular target's **thermal relaxation time (TRT)** is useful in clinical practice to pick the correct pulse duration. TRT is simply defined as the time required for substantial cooling of the target structure. TRT is strongly related to target size, and this variation accounts for the wide range of laser pulse durations needed for optimal dermatological lasers. A simple and useful approximation is that $TRT \approx d^2$, when TRT is in units of seconds, and d is the target size in millimeters. For example, a 1 mm leg vein cools in about 1 second, while a 0.2 mm telangiectasia, typical for rosacea, cools in about 0.04 seconds (40 ms), and a 0.03 mm venule in a child's port-wine stain cools in about 0.001 seconds (1 ms). The optimal laser or IPL pulse duration is typically about equal to the TRT. In this example, a very long exposure from a low-power KTP (532 nm) laser would be appropriate for treating the leg vein. A higher power KTP or pulsed dye (595 nm) laser operated at about 20–40 ms would be appropriate for the rosacea-associated telangiectasia, and a pulsed dye laser operated at about 1 ms would be appropriate for the pediatric port-wine stain. This extreme dependence of TRT on target size applies all the way down to the nanoscale of subcellular targets. Q-switched lasers are used in dermatology because their 10–100 nanosecond pulse durations are shorter than the TRT for targets such as tattoo ink particles, melanosomes, and drug pigmentation deposits (see Case study 1).

The matching of TRT and pulse duration is clinically important to achieve efficacy, avoid side effects, and even to define the targets that will respond. For example, consider a young man with both nevus of Ota and a dark beard on his face. Both the nevus and his beard hair contain high concentrations of the same chromophore, melanin. A Q-switched alexandrite laser (~755 nm wavelength) will be highly effective for fading his nevus of Ota, because the targets are small, isolated melanocytes scattered deeply throughout his dermis. The appropriate end point is immediate whitening, due to microscopic gas bubbles formed when the target melanocytes in his dermis are fractured. However, this Q-switched alexandrite laser will not permanently remove his hair, because its pulse duration is a million times shorter than the TRT for a terminal hair follicle. This laser merely vaporizes the hair shaft (which is already dead) before heat can flow to the hair follicle epithelium and the patient can be informed with confidence that his beard will not be accidentally removed.

In contrast, a long-pulse (3–30 ms) alexandrite laser *at the identical wavelength* could permanently remove his beard without affecting his nevus of Ota. This long pulse duration is incapable of providing thermal confinement in something as small as an isolated melanocyte, but allows plenty of time for heating of the entire hair follicle without vaporizing its pigmented hair shaft.

A common professional liability issue related to pulse duration is the use of long-pulsed sources such as IPLs, broadly available for laser hair removal, for the treatment of tattoos. Long-pulsed lasers and IPLs emit millisecond domain pulses that heat the tattooed skin at large instead of the individual ink particles, because the pulse duration greatly exceeds the TRT of the ink particle. The surrounding dermis is therefore heated causing unselective thermal damage, blistering, dyschromia and scarring, as reported by Wenzel and co-workers in 2009. Unfortunately, similar mistakes are commonly observed due to the lack of a full understanding of SP and incorrect choice of treatment pulse width.

The third factor for optimal SP is sufficient fluence to affect the targets. In general, the fluence necessary is inversely related to absorption by the target structures – stronger absorption requires lower fluence, and vice versa. This is the reason, for example, that a typical alexandrite laser fluence for treatment of a port-wine stain (see **Case study 2**) is 40 J/cm^2, while that for pulsed dye laser treatment of the same lesion may be only 8 J/cm^2.

CASE STUDY 2
The Tindal Effect

A 6-year-old child with Sturge-Weber syndrome has a large port-wine stain on her arm. She has been treated with 595 nm pulsed dye laser, but after 10 sessions the lesion seems unresponsive to treatment. Another dermatologist starts treatment with a 755 nm long-pulse alexandrite laser and, unlike the previous treatment, the lesion seems to respond quite well.

For pulsed sources, it is not uncommon to see frequency as one of the parameters. Frequency is the measurement of repetition rate of a laser pulse in a given period of time (seconds) and is measured in hertz (Hz), where 1 Hz is 1 pulse/second. It is useful to use higher repetition rates for treatments that require a large number of laser pulses (e.g. large tattoos). Although it is tedious to treat a large tattoo using 1 pulse/second, increasing the frequency of pulses makes the treatment less time consuming (and more challenging to distribute the pulses uniformly).

Skin cooling: limiting thermal damage to the intended targets

Sparing of the epidermis and superficial dermis is important for selective destruction of deeper structures and can be improved by the use of appropriate skin cooling.

Cooling can be applied before (pre-cooling), during (parallel cooling), and after the laser pulse (post-cooling). Similarly to laser-induced tissue heating, cooling should be applied keeping in mind the histological target. According to Zenzie et al, the greater the depth of an anatomical structure, the longer the cooling should be applied. For epidermal protection, Sakamoto and co-workers reported that 20–50 ms is enough, while for epidermal and dermal protection (e.g. for targeting subcutaneous fat) cooling should be applied for 5–10 seconds. Cooling can be applied using direct solid contact cooling (e.g. cold sapphire window), automated cryogen spray (DCD™, direct cooling devices) or by blowing direct cold air. Cold-air cooling has the advantage of bulk skin cooling, which limits pain, edema, and the risk of burns from residual heat.

For the choice of proper dosimetry, it is crucial to be familiar with the particular device being used, and to carefully observe skin response to treatment. The combination of laser wavelength, pulse duration, spot size, skin cooling, and dosimetry can suggest initial treatment parameters, but only careful observation of immediate clinical end points will ensure efficacy (Figs 1.3–1.5), helping to avoid side effects. Common clinical end points are summarized in Table 1.1.

Pearl 6

Cooling is mandatory to protect the epidermis and superficial dermis during selective photothermolysis.

Pearl 7

Careful examination of immediate skin end points can help in choosing laser parameters.

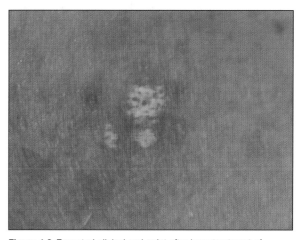

Figure 1.3 Expected clinical end point after laser treatment of pigmented lesions using a Q-switched 755 nm alexandrite laser for solar lentigines. Immediate response observed with epidermal whitening due to steam bubbles.

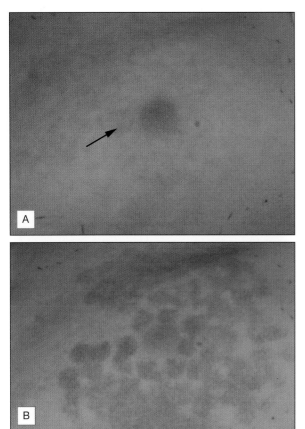

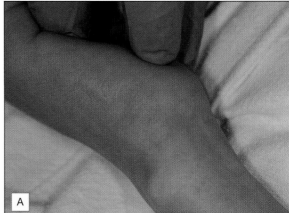

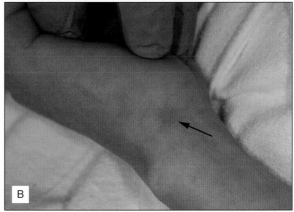

Figure 1.4 Expected clinical end point after laser treatment of a vascular lesion: (**A**) Child's chest with port-wine stain previously treated with laser, before PDL session, with immediate response after a single 585 nm pulsed-dye laser pulse, 3 ms pulse width, 6 mm spot size, 9 J/cm² with dynamic cooling (arrow). (**B**) Note immediate round-shaped purpura where laser is applied, indicating vessel coagulation.

Figure 1.5 Expected clinical end point after laser treatment of a vascular lesion: (**A**) Wrist with port-wine stain. (**B**) Immediate response after a single (arrow) 755 nm alexandrite laser pulse, 1.5 ms pulse width, 6 mm spot size, 80 J/cm² with dynamic cooling. Note immediate bluish color, indicating vessel coagulation.

Pearl 8

Side effects are usually a consequence of poor choice of light source and parameters.

Fractional photothermolysis

Fractional photothermolysis (FP) uses microbeams of laser to target the tissue, inducing microthermal zones (MTZ) of injury, as reported by Manstein and colleagues in 2004. Each MTZ is typically 100–300 µm in diameter. The depth and density (number per unit area) of the microlaser beams applied to the tissue can be adjusted depending on the clinical indication. The advantage of this technique is that it spares untreated skin surrounding each MTZ, allowing fast healing and reducing the risk of side effects. A typical FP treatment session provides laser exposure to about 10–50% of the skin.

Soon after its introduction in 2004, the concept of FP has been widely embraced in dermatology. A number of new devices, laser wavelengths, and clinical indications have been developed with success. In principle, FP can be applied with a wide variety of energy sources capable of producing an array of small zones of skin damage. These include various non-ablative NIR lasers (1320–1550 nm; 1927 nm thulium) and ablative lasers (2940 nm erbium; 10600 nm CO_2). Currently, even visible light and other technologies such as ultrasound and radiofrequency devices have been using fractionated applicators. Photoaging and pigmentary alterations, scar treatment, melasma, striae, and xanthelasma are examples of the variety of clinical indications that can be treated with FP (see respectively the studies by Manstein et al, Alster et al, Tannous & Astner, Kim et al and Katz et al).

Interestingly, in addition to local thermal destruction and stimulation, fractionated devices may also play an important role for drug delivery into the tissue and for extruding material out of the skin, as in the studies by Haedersdal et al. This has also been recently reported by Ibrahimi et al using an ablative fractionated erbium:YAG laser to treat an allergic tattoo reaction with success.

Table 1.1 Most common laser types used in dermatology

Primary chromophores	Lasers	Wavelength (nm)	Mode/pulse width range	Typical applications	Expected clinical end points	Unwanted end points
N/A	Excimer	308	QCW (ns pulses)	UVB phototherapy of psoriasis; vitiligo; atopic dermatitis	Non-selective damage with erythema, mild edema	
Hemoglobin	Pulsed dye (yellow)	577–600	Pulsed 0.45–1.5 ms; 10–40 ms stuttered	Especially PWS; telangiectasia; warts; red scars; mild photodamage	Purpura, durable vessel darkening, vessel disappearance, selective coagulation	Selective photothermolysis should NEVER present: ablation, uniform gray coagulation, positive Nikolski sign, shrinkage or darkening of normal skin (e.g. chrysiasis)
Hemoglobin, melanin	KTP	532	QCW, CW, or pulsed	Telangiectasia; benign lentigo; warts		
Melanin, hemoglobin, water (weak)	Xenon flashlamp (IPL)	500–1200	Pulsed 2–50 ms; 20–100 ms stuttered or single pulse	Telangiectasia; mild photodamage; hair removal; benign lentigo	Subtle darkening of pigmented lesions, vessel disappearance	
Melanin, hemoglobin (weak)	Long-pulsed alexandrite	755	Pulsed 1.5–40.0 ms stuttered	Hair removal; leg veins; hypertrophic PWS	Perifollicular erythema, edema at 5 minutes	
Melanin	Long-pulsed ruby	694	Pulsed 3 ms; 100 ms stuttered	Hair removal; some nevi		
Melanin	Diode	800	Pulsed 5–500 ms	Hair removal; venous lakes, telangiectasias, leg veins		
Melanin	Long-pulsed Nd:YAG	1064	Pulsed or stuttered, 3–100 ms	Hair removal in dark skin; leg veins		
Melanin and tattoos	Q-switched Nd:YAG	532 1064	Q-switched 5–10 ns	532: Epidermal pigment; red tattoos 1064: Epidermal/dermal pigment (lentigines, nevus of Ota, etc.); tattoos (black 1064, red 532)	Immediate whitening	
Melanin and tattoos (except red)	Q-switched ruby	694	Q-switched 20 ns	Epidermal/dermal pigment; lentigines, nevus of Ota; tattoos (black, blue, green)		
Melanin and tattoos (except red)	Q-switched alexandrite	755	Q-switched 50–100 ns	Epidermal/dermal pigment; lentigines, nevus of Ota; tattoos (black, blue, green)		
Water	Mid-IR Nd:YAG	1320	Pulsed 20–50 ms stuttered macropulses	Non-ablative dermal remodeling	Non-selective damage: erythema, edema, sometimes pinpoint bleeding	
Water	Mid-IR diode	1450	Pulsed 5–260 ms	Non-ablative dermal remodeling, fractional resurfacing		

Continued

Table 1.1 Most common laser types used in dermatology—cont'd

Primary chromophores	Lasers	Wavelength (nm)	Mode/pulse width range	Typical applications	Expected clinical end points	Unwanted end points
Water	Erbium:glass	1540	Pulsed 1–10 ms	Non-ablative dermal remodeling, acne, fractional resurfacing		
Water	Thulium:YAG	1927	Pulsed 10 ms	Non-ablative/ablative dermal remodeling, acne, fractional resurfacing		
Water	Erbium:YAG	2940	Pulsed 0.1–3 ms	Ablation of epidermal lesions; skin resurfacing; ablative fractional resurfacing		
Water	CO_2	10600	CW, scanned or pulsed/1 μs–1 ms	Ablation of lesions; resurfacing for moderate – severe photodamage; rhytides; scars, ablative fractional resurfacing		

CW: continuous wave; QCW: quasi-continuous wave (a rapid low-energy pulse train); pulsed: high-energy pulses; PWS: port-wine stain; PDL: pulsed dye laser; IPL: intense pulsed light; SP: selective photothermolysis.

Whereas conventional treatment of allergic tattoo reactions with a Q-switched laser alone could likely increase immunogenicity of the tattoo pigment post-treatment and the risk of a systemic allergic response, the ablative fractional laser has shown the ability to remove allergic tattoo pigment as an alternative method without inducing a systemic allergic reaction.

Pearl 9

Fractional photothermolysis can be performed with ablative and non-ablative energy sources.

Conclusion

It is likely that fractional photothermolysis lasers and similar fractional treatment technology will continue to evolve into unforeseen applications. Many interesting, fundamental, and clinically important questions remain to be answered about lasers in dermatology.

Further reading

Alster TS, Tanzi EL, Lazarus M, et al 2007 The use of fractional laser photothermolysis for the treatment of atrophic scars. Dermatologic Surgery 33(3):295-299

Anderson RR, Farinelli W, Laubach H, et al 2006 Selective photothermolysis of lipid-rich tissues: a free electron laser study. Lasers in Surgery and Medicine 38(10):913-919

Anderson RR, Parrish JA 1983 Selective photothermolysis: precise microsurgery by selective absorption of pulsed radiation. Science 220(4596):524-527

Chang CJ, Nelson JS 1999 Cryogen spray cooling and higher fluence pulsed dye laser treatment improve port-wine stain clearance while minimizing epidermal damage. Dermatologic Surgery 25(10):767-772

Grossman MC, Dierickx C, Farinelli W, et al 1996 Damage to hair follicles by normal-mode ruby laser pulses. Journal of the American Academy of Dermatology 35(6):889-894

Haedersdal M, Katsnelson J, Sakamoto FH, et al 2011 Enhanced uptake and photoactivation of topical methyl aminolevulinate after fractional CO2 laser pretreatment. Lasers in Surgery and Medicine 43(8):804-813

Haedersdal M, Sakamoto FH, Farinelli WA, et al 2010 Fractional CO(2) laser-assisted drug delivery. Lasers in Surgery and Medicine 42(2):113-122

Ibrahimi OA, Syed Z, Sakamoto FH, et al 2011 Treatment of tattoo allergy with ablative fractional resurfacing: a novel paradigm for tattoo removal. Journal of the American Academy of Dermatology 64(6):1111-1114

Izikson L, Nelson JS, Anderson RR, et al 2009 Treatment of hypertrophic and resistant port wine stains with a 755 nm laser: a case series of 20 patients. Lasers in Surgery and Medicine 41(6):427-432

Katz TM, Goldberg LH, Friedman PM, et al 2009 Fractional photothermolysis: a new therapeutic modality for xanthelasma. Archives of Dermatology 145(10):1091-1094

Kim BJ, Lee DH, Kim MN, et al 2008 Fractional photothermolysis for the treatment of striae distensae in Asian skin. American Journal of Clinical Dermatology 9(1):33-37

Manstein D, Herron GS, Sink RK, et al 2004 Fractional photothermolysis: a new concept for cutaneous remodeling using microscopic patterns of thermal injury. Lasers in Surgery and Medicine 34(5):426-438

Sakamoto FH, Doukas AG, Farinelli WA, et al 2012 Selective photothermolysis to target sebaceous glands: Theoretical estimation of parameters and preliminary results using a free electron laser. Lasers in Surgery and Medicine 44(2):175-183

Sakamoto FH, Wall T, et al 2007 Lasers and flashlamps in dermatology. In: Wolff K, Goldsmith LA, Katzet SI, et al (eds) Fitzpatrick's dermatology in general medicine vol II. The McGraw-Hill Companies, Inc., Columbus, p 2263-2279

Tannous ZS, Astner S 2005 Utilizing fractional resurfacing in the treatment of therapy-resistant melasma. Journal of Cosmetic Laser Therapy 7(1):39-43

Wenzel S, Landthaler M, Baumler W, et al 2009 Recurring mistakes in tattoo removal. A case series. Dermatology 218(2):164-167

Zenzie HH, Altshuler GB, Smirnov MZ, et al 2000 Evaluation of cooling methods for laser dermatology. Lasers in Surgery and Medicine 26(2):130-144

2

Laser treatment of vascular lesions

Iris Kedar Rubin, Kristen M. Kelly

Summary and Key Features

- Vascular lesions are one of the most common indications for laser treatment
- Treatment of vascular lesions implements the theory of selective photothermolysis, confining thermal injury to the target of interest
- Pulsed dye laser remains the gold standard treatment for port-wine stains, and while most improve, the minority clear completely
- Early laser treatment improves port-wine stain response
- Alexandrite laser can be implemented for treatment of hypertrophic, or pulsed dye laser resistant, port-wine stains
- Indications for laser treatment of hemangiomas includes ulcerated lesions and involuted lesions with residual telangiectasias and/or textural change
- The role of laser treatment for proliferating hemangiomas remains less clear, and may be most beneficial for superficial hemangiomas
- Deeper-penetrating near-infrared lasers may be implemented to treat select venous malformations
- Vascular lasers and intense pulsed light are the treatment of choice for the background erythema and telangiectasias associated with rosacea
- Poikiloderma of Civatte can be successfully treated with intense pulsed light, or a combination of vascular and pigment selective lasers

Introduction and history

One of the first applications of lasers in dermatology was the removal of vascular lesions. Laser surgery has become the treatment of choice for many vascular lesions. The most common indications for treatment are vascular anomalies including port-wine stain birthmarks (PWS) and hemangiomas, as well as facial erythema and telangiectasias. Vascular specific lasers have seen an evolution from the historically used continuous wave lasers to pulsed lasers that implement the theory of selective photothermolysis, introduced by Anderson and Parrish in 1983.

In 1961, Dr Leon Goldman pioneered the use of lasers with a ruby device. Argon lasers were developed later in the 1960s and improved the color of PWS and hemangiomas, but resulted in unacceptably high rates of scarring and depigmentation due to non-specific heating of the superficial dermis. The theory of selective photothermolysis provided a mechanism to confine thermal injury to the target of interest and minimize collateral damage to surrounding tissue and allowed development of pulsed lasers.

Three components are necessary for selective photothermolysis: (1) a laser wavelength with preferential absorption of the target chromophore, (2) appropriate pulse duration matched to the target size, and (3) a fluence that both treats the target and minimizes non-specific thermal related injury. The ideal pulse duration is equal to or somewhat shorter than the thermal relaxation time of the target vessel. The thermal relaxation time is defined as the time for 50% of the heat to dissipate from the target of interest. A pulse duration that is too short may not be effective, whereas one that is too long may cause heat to dissipate to surrounding structures and cause unwanted thermal injury. The classic target chromophore for vascular lesions has been oxyhemoglobin, which has the greatest absorption peaks at 418, 542, and 577 nm (Fig. 2.1). The laser light is absorbed by oxyhemoglobin, and converted to heat, which is transferred to the vessel wall causing coagulation and vessel closure. Other hemoglobin species have more recently been recognized as appropriate targets, depending on the vascular lesion. For example, venous lesions may benefit from wavelengths of light that target deoxyhemoglobin. The alexandrite laser at 755 nm is close to a deoxyhemoglobin absorption peak and has been used for refractory or hypertrophic PWS, a venocapillary malformation. Methemoglobin absorption has also been recognized as a potential target chromophore.

Pulsed dye lasers (PDL) became available in 1986, and were initially developed at 577 nm to target the yellow absorption peak of oxyhemoglobin. It was later realized that, for selective photothermolysis to occur, the laser wavelength did not have to be at an absorption peak for the target chromophore as long as preferential absorption

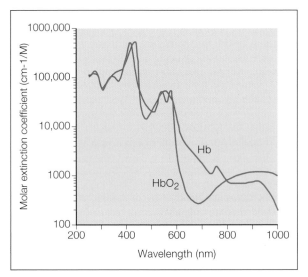

Figure 2.1 Optical absorption of hemoglobin. *Source: Dr Scott Prahl, http://omlc.ogi.edu/spectra/hemoglobin.*

Table 2.1 Comparison of infantile hemangioma and port-wine stain

	Infantile hemangioma	Port-wine stain
Onset	▪ First few weeks of life ▪ Precursor may be present at birth	▪ Present at birth
Course	▪ Proliferative period in first year of life, followed by slow involution	▪ Does not regress ▪ May become hypertrophic, more violaceous with age ▪ May develop vascular blebs
Tissue marker	▪ GLUT1 positive	▪ GLUT1 negative

was still present. PDLs shifted to 585 nm, allowing for a depth of penetration of approximately 1.16 mm; 595 nm PDLs later became available to achieve greater depth of penetration. PDLs have also evolved to incorporate longer pulse durations. Early PDLs had a fixed pulse duration of 0.45 ms, whereas currently available PDLs have pulse durations from 0.45–40 ms. Longer pulse durations have the advantage of treating without purpura.

Epidermal cooling was introduced in the 1990s as a means to protect the epidermis, minimizing pigmentary changes and scarring. Cooling also permits the utilization of higher fluences and thus provides greater treatment efficacy. In addition, cooling minimizes discomfort associated with treatment. Modern cooling devices include dynamic spray, contact, and forced cold-air cooling.

Since the PDL penetrates to a depth of only 1–2 mm, other lasers have been developed to treat vascular lesions in an attempt to achieve a greater depth of penetration. The alexandrite laser at 755 nm and neodymium:yttrium aluminum garnet (Nd:YAG) laser at 1064 nm, for example, penetrate up to 50–75% deeper into the skin. Given that the absolute absorption of hemoglobin species is lower at these wavelengths, higher fluences are required.

Intense pulsed light (IPL) devices emit polychromatic non-coherent broadband light from 420 to 1400 nm with varying pulse durations. Filters are implemented to remove unwanted shorter wavelengths of light to treat vascular lesions with blue-green to yellow wavelengths.

The most commonly used vascular lasers and light sources include:

▪ PDLs (585 nm, 595 nm)
▪ potassium titanyl phosphate (KTP) (532 nm)
▪ near-infrared long-pulsed lasers: alexandrite (755 nm), diode (800–810 nm, 940 nm), and Nd:YAG (1064 nm)
▪ dual-wavelength lasers: Cynergy by Cynosure (pulsed dye at 595 nm and Nd:YAG at 1064 nm)
▪ IPL sources with appropriate vascular-specific filters.

Vascular anomalies classification

The International Society for the Study of Vascular Anomalies (ISSVA) adopted a classification system in 1996 with two main categories. Vascular tumors are characterized by a proliferation of blood vessels, infantile hemangiomas being the most common. Vascular malformations are characterized by vessels with abnormal structure and normal endothelial cell turnover. Vascular malformations can be further subdivided into slow-flow lesions and fast-flow lesions. Capillary malformations, venous malformations, and lymphatic malformations are slow-flow lesions. Arterial malformations and arteriovenous malformations are fast-flow lesions. Complex-combined vascular malformations occur as well.

PWS, a type of capillary malformation, and hemangiomas are the two most common vascular anomalies that present for laser treatment (Table 2.1).

Port-wine stain birthmarks

Overview

PWS are vascular malformations that are composed of ectatic capillaries and post-capillary venules in the superficial vascular plexus. PWS vessels are characterized by diminished vascular tone and decreased density of nerves, especially those with autonomic function. In most cases, PWS are congenital, though in rare cases they may be acquired. PWS are found in approximately 0.3% of newborns. They tend to occur on the head and neck, although they may appear anywhere on the body. PWS persist throughout life and many thicken with time (Fig. 2.2). Geronemus et al reported that the mean age of

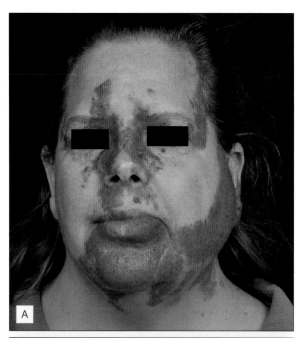

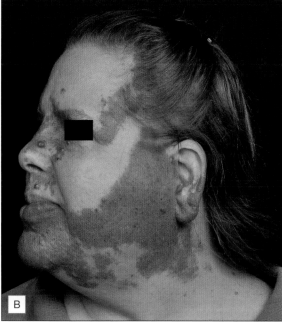

Figure 2.2 (**A**, **B**) Hypertrophic port-wine stain not yet treated.

PWS can be associated with various syndromes that are important to identify. A PWS in the V1 distribution raises the question of Sturge-Weber syndrome (SWS), which may have associated glaucoma, seizures, and developmental delay. Klippel-Trenaunay syndrome involves a PWS on an extremity, limb hypertrophy, and associated lymphatic/venous malformations. PWS can also occur in association with arteriovenous malformations in capillary malformation/arteriovenous malformation syndrome.

The goal of treatment of a PWS is to decrease or eliminate the red or sometimes violaceous color, improve appearance, and diminish psychosocial discomfort caused by these lesions. Treatment may also prevent development of blebs that may bleed or become infected. It has been theorized that treating PWS early may prevent hypertrophy as well. The PDL, which is strongly absorbed by oxyhemoglobin, is the most commonly used laser for treatment. Although PDL is effective and approximately 80% improve with treatment, only about 20% of PWS clear completely. Deeper-penetrating lasers have been used in an attempt to improve treatment outcomes. PWS response to laser treatment is variable. A study by Nguyen et al found predictors of improved response include small size (<20 cm^2), location over bony areas, in particular the central forehead, and early treatment. A retrospective study by Chapas et al of 49 infants who started laser treatment by the age of 6 months demonstrated an impressive average clearance of 88.6% after 1 year, suggesting that early treatment may be advisable. Early treatment may be more beneficial due to thinner lesions and overall smaller lesions. Other factors must be considered in deciding when to initiate treatment, including anesthesia and the associated risks and benefits.

Huikeshoven et al have shown that PWS may redarken after laser therapy, though recurrent areas are still significantly lighter compared with baseline. This occurrence of redarkening may be due to revascularization that occurs as a response to injury and hypoxia and/or progressive dilatation of residual vessels as a result of decreased autonomic nerves.

Treatment

The PDL is the most commonly used laser to treat PWS. Treatments are typically done at 4–6 week intervals, and it is not uncommon for 10 or more treatments to be performed initially until a plateau is reached or the lesion clears (Fig. 2.3). Larger spot sizes allow for greater depth of penetration and so the clinician should select the largest spot size that will provide sufficient fluence to achieve the desired end point, while confining the treatment to the area of interest. It is advisable to determine the fluence threshold on the darkest portion of the PWS with 1 or 2 test pulses before treating the entire lesion. The fluence is adjusted to achieve the desired end point. For the PDL, the desired end point is immediate purpura. A confluent gray color signifies that the fluence is too high. A cookbook approach to treatment may result in complications.

hypertrophy is 37 years and, by the fifth decade, approximately 65% of lesions had become hypertrophied or nodular. There may be associated soft tissue overgrowth, leading to functional impairment in areas such as the lip or eyelid. Vascular blebs often form and may bleed with minimal trauma. These lesions are often considered disfiguring and many patients or their families seek treatment. PWS vessels vary in size from 7–300 μm with older patients tending to have larger vessels.

Changing the pulse duration may allow targeting of different-sized vessels and can be useful. Dierickx et al identified the ideal pulse duration for PWS treatment to be 1–10 ms. In practice, treatment often begins at 1.5 ms, though this may be adjusted down to 0.45 ms and up to 6 ms. Parameters to consider include 7–10 mm spot size, pulse duration of 0.45–6 ms, and fluence of 5.5–9.5 J/cm^2 with appropriate epidermal cooling. Lower energies are used for larger spot sizes, with shorter pulse durations, and in patients with darker skin types. Longer pulse durations are advisable in darker skin types. Treatment should start at lower energies and this can be increased if treatments are tolerated well. Parameters vary by device.

Pearl 3

Proper cooling is essential to protect the epidermis and minimize side effects, i.e. scarring and pigmentary changes.

Prior to treatment, it is helpful to outline the borders of the PWS as laser pulses or topical anesthesia can induce erythema that can blur the border. Surgilube may be placed on eyebrows and eyelashes to avoid singeing. Although hair often regrows, permanent hair loss can occur on eyelashes at any age with PDL treatment, given the close proximity of the follicles to the surface. In addition, permanent hair loss can occur on the eyebrows and scalp of young children, in particular those with dark hair.

Pearl 4

Outline PWS borders prior to treatment, as laser pulses can induce erythema that blurs the border. The PWS may be outlined with a marking pen, or with purpuric laser pulses at the start of treatment.

When treating darker skin types, the risk of hypopigmentation and hyperpigmentation can be minimized by using appropriate cooling and longer pulse durations. Treatment intervals may need to be longer to allow for any pigmentation changes to resolve before proceeding with additional treatment. Care must be taken with leg lesions as legs are prone to hyperpigmentation.

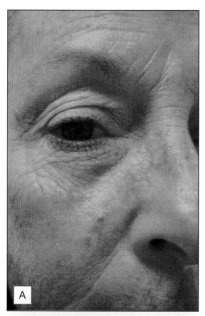

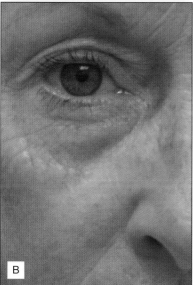

Figure 2.3 Port-wine stain: (**A**) pre and (**B**) post pulsed dye laser treatments.

Pearl 1

Larger spot sizes increase the depth of penetration. For the PDL, treat with the largest spot that will provide adequate fluence and confine the treatment to the area of interest.

Pearl 2

Larger spot sizes produce less scatter of light and may require lower fluences.

Pearl 5

Know, follow, and trust the desired clinical treatment end point, not a setting number.

Use longer pulse durations and/or lower fluences for darker skin.

The alexandrite laser is typically used for PDL-resistant lesions, though it may be implemented as a first-line treatment for hypertrophic violaceous lesions in adults (Fig. 2.4). The end point is a subtle gray-blue discoloration followed by deeper purpura that takes several minutes to develop. A sustained gray color indicates that the fluence is too high, and there is a risk of scarring. Care must be

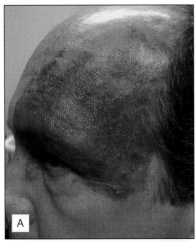

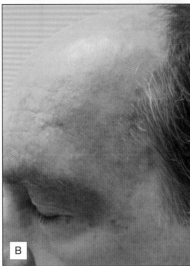

Figure 2.4 Violaceous, hypertrophic port-wine stain: (**A**) pre and (**B**) post alexandrite laser treatments. Note improvement in color and thickness. *Courtesy of Dr Rox Anderson.*

taken not to overlap pulses as scarring can occur. Note that the range of appropriate fluences for alexandrite laser use is quite broad.

The Nd:YAG laser and combined 595, 1064 nm lasers can also be used for PWS. Although depth of penetration can be increased, there is a narrow therapeutic window with these devices and caution is advised owing to the risk of scarring. It is recommended that these devices be used only by experienced laser surgeons. IPL treatment with appropriate vascular filters has also been reported to be effective for treatment of PWS. Treatment with any of the near-infrared lasers, or IPL, in hair-bearing areas may lead to permanent hair loss.

Treatment of associated vascular nodules can be done by excision or laser. PDL may be used, though several pulses may be required. Stack pulsing can be used, but should be approached cautiously as risk of injury will be increased. Given the limited depth of penetration of PDL, near-infrared lasers such as the alexandrite and Nd:YAG lasers may be necessary. CO_2 and Er:YAG lasers have also been utilized to successfully ablate nodules.

Photodynamic therapy (PDT) has been utilized successfully to treat PWS, primarily in China. Use of systemically administered hematoporphyrin photosensitizers results in prolonged photosensitivity (weeks), which limits use. Alternative photosensitizers, such as benzoporphyrin derivative monoacid ring A and mono-L-aspartyl chlorin e6 (Npe6), have shorter periods of photosensitivity and may offer promising alternatives. PDT may potentially be a useful treatment if parameters can be optimized. Combined photodynamic therapies and PDL has been studied and may improve safety. Recently there has been great interest in improving treatment efficacy by combining light-based removal of PWS with post-treatment anti-angiogenic agents. This approach is currently experimental, but is promising.

Infantile hemangiomas

Overview

Hemangiomas of infancy are benign endothelial cell proliferations that represent the most common tumor of infancy occurring in 4–10% of infants. Hemangiomas occur more often in girls, with a 3:1 predominance, and 60% occur on the head and neck. Hemangiomas typically present within the first 4 weeks of age. There may be an early macular stain present at birth that is hypopigmented, red, or telangiectatic. Hemangiomas have been theorized to be derived from embolized placental stem cells. Recently it has been proposed that hemangiomas may arise as a response to tissue hypoxia. Hemangiomas express GLUT1, differentiating them from other vascular tumors and vascular malformations. GLUT1 is a fetal-type endothelial glucose transporter. Hemangiomas may be characterized as localized or segmental, and as superficial (clinically red), deep (clinically blue or skin colored) or mixed.

The proliferative period typically lasts until 6–8 months for superficial hemangiomas, though deep hemangiomas may proliferate longer. Involution then occurs more slowly over years. Approximately 50% of hemangiomas have regressed by age 5 and 90% have regressed by age 9. After regression, many hemangiomas leave behind residual fibrofatty tissue, atrophy, and/or telangiectasias.

Hemangiomas typically do not require imaging studies. Multiple hemangiomas or hemangiomas in certain locations may prompt radiologic investigation to assess for possible associated syndromes. PHACES syndrome must be considered in large segmental facial hemangiomas and is characterized by **p**osterior fossa malformations, **h**emangiomas, **a**rterial anomalies, **c**oarctation of the aorta, **e**ye abnormalities, and **s**ternal or **s**upraumbilical raphe. Perineal hemangiomas may prompt an evaluation for PELVIS syndrome: **p**erineal hemangioma, **e**xternal genital malformations, lipomyelomeningocele, vesicorenal abnormalities, imperforate anus, and skin tags. Diffuse neonatal hemangiomatosis involves multiple skin hemangiomas and signifies a risk of visceral hemangiomas, most commonly liver followed by the gastrointestinal tract.

Two rare types of hemangiomas that are present at birth and are GLUT1 negative include non-involuting congential hemangiomas (NICH) and rapidly involuting congential hemangiomas (RICH).

Treatment

Treatment of hemangiomas is indicated for functional impairment, as well as for complications such as ulceration, infection, or bleeding. Hemangiomas can cause functional difficulties when critical anatomical structures are affected, including airway compromise, symptomatic hepatic involvement, visual obstruction, or auditory canal obstruction.

The historic treatment for many hemangiomas, in the absence of functional difficulties or complications, has been to 'watch and wait', so-called active non-intervention. More recently it has been recognized that an indication for treatment is prevention of long-term scarring. Early treatment of hemangiomas may help minimize the scarring associated with hemangiomas, and the psychosocial distress that can occur with the watch and wait approach. Hemangiomas on the nose, lips, glabella, and on the chest in females, may be considered cosmetically sensitive.

Hemangioma treatment is tailored on an individual patient basis, taking into account the extent of the lesion, depth, and degree of functional impairment. Treatment options include topical treatments, intralesional corticosteroids, systemic medications, laser, and surgical excision. A combination approach can be helpful.

Topical treatments are most useful for superficial hemangiomas, and include high-potency topical corticosteroids, topical timolol (a beta blocker recently reported to be effective, initially in superficial eyelid hemangiomas), and possibly imiquimod, though efficacy has been limited and is controversial. Topical becaplermin gel, a recombinant platelet-derived growth factor, can expedite healing of ulcerated lesions. Ulcerated lesions may also be treated with local wound care, topical antibiotics, barrier creams, and occlusive dressings.

Oral treatments may be indicated for functional impairment, complications such as significant ulceration, or hemangiomas with potential for significant disfigurement. Traditionally the most commonly implemented oral treatment for hemangiomas was corticosteroids. More recently, oral propranolol, a beta blocker, has been found to improve hemangiomas. Although useful, systemic treatments have potential side effects. Systemic corticosteroids can cause irritability, gastric upset, transient growth retardation, adrenal suppression, and immunosuppression with rare reports of pneumonia. Though generally well tolerated, potential side effects with propranolol include hypoglycemia, bronchospasm, hyperkalemia, hypotension, and

bradycardia. Interferon alpha was used to treat hemangiomas, though it has fallen out of favor owing to the relatively high frequency of spastic diplegia, a potentially devastating consequence. Vincristine, a chemotherapeutic agent, has been used in refractory and life-threatening cases.

The role of laser in the proliferative and involuting stages is not clear and remains controversial. Laser treatment during the proliferative period is advocated by some, with the goal of halting further growth and accelerating involution. Laser treatment is most effective for superficial hemangiomas given the laser light's limited depth of penetration. For mixed superficial and deep lesions, PDL may be implemented to lighten the color, though it will not affect the deeper component. There has yet to be a well-designed controlled study confirming the benefits of early laser treatment for uncomplicated hemangiomas. One commonly cited randomized and controlled study by Batta et al compared early PDL treatment with no treatment and found early clearance with PDL, though at 1 year there was no difference in residual hemangioma. Side effects from laser treatment including skin atrophy and hypopigmentation were seen, likely due to lack of cooling that is present on modern PDLs.

A range of fluences has been used for PDL treatment of proliferating hemangiomas. Risks of laser treatment include ulceration that can result in scarring; in our opinion, proliferating lesions should be approached cautiously with lower fluences. Treatment settings to consider for PDL include pulse duration 0.45–1.5 ms, 10 or 7 mm spot, fluence 4–7 J/cm^2, and appropriate skin cooling. Lower fluences and longer pulse durations are advisable in darker skin types. Parameters vary by device. Multiple treatments are generally required, and may be done at 2-week intervals for rapidly proliferating lesions or 4–6-week intervals for involuting lesions. The main risks of treatment are ulceration and scarring, as well as hypopigmentation. There have been rare reports of serious bleeding after PDL treatment for hemangiomas, primarily with older lasers without cooling, and one case with a 595 nm laser with cooling, using relatively high fluences (12 J/cm^2).

There is general agreement that PDL is effective for the treatment of ulcerated hemangiomas. A study by David et al of 78 patients with ulcerated hemangiomas showed that 91% improved after a mean of two PDL treatments. Laser treatment may also be beneficial for hemangiomas in areas prone to ulceration, specifically the anogenital area.

Laser treatment of involuted lesions is also commonly accepted. PDL is beneficial for the residual telangiectasia associated with involuted hemangiomas, and fractionated non-ablative and ablative lasers can improve texture of residual fibrofatty tissue.

The KTP laser and IPL have also been implemented to successfully treat hemangiomas. Some have utilized the Nd:YAG laser for hemangiomas in order to get greater depth of penetration. The longer wavelength also has less competing melanin absorption. Extreme caution is required as there is a narrow therapeutic window for Nd:YAG treatment and significant ulceration and scarring can easily occur.

Venous malformations

Venous malformations present clinically as soft, compressible, non-pulsatile blue-violaceous papules or nodules that increase in size with measures that increase venous pressure, such as the dependent position. Vessel walls may exhibit calcifications, and phleboliths are considered pathognomonic. Venous malformations are slow-flow lesions that may be present at birth, or present later in life as they progress. MRI imaging for larger lesion is advised to assess the extent of the lesion.

Laser treatment can be indicated for small and discrete venous malformations, for example on the lip (Fig. 2.5). The goal is to decrease the size of lesion and at times complete clearance may be possible, though venous malformations have a tendency for recanalization. Multiple treatment modalities are used for larger lesions including surgery and sclerotherapy. Laser treatment may also be performed for larger venous malformations with the goal of debulking prior to surgery. Laser treatment of venous malformations requires a deeper penetrating laser, and the near-infrared lasers, specifically diode or Nd:YAG, are most commonly implemented. Treatment of these lesions is complex and best handled by experienced surgeons. Scherer and Waner described the benefits of Nd:YAG laser therapy for complex venous malformations including

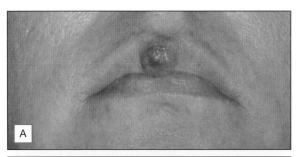

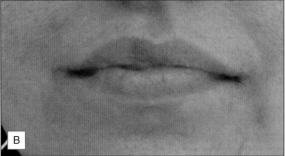

Figure 2.5 Venous malformation: (**A**) pre and (**B**) post diode laser treatments. There is significant reduction in size and improvement in color. Patient was undergoing further treatments. *Courtesy of Dr Rox Anderson.*

tissue shrinkage, improved color, and induction of dermal fibrosis, thus reducing the risk of skin loss in surgery and sclerotherapy. In their hands, swelling lasted approximately 2 weeks, and blistering, dyspigmentation, and scarring occurred in <5% of patients.

Other vascular malformations

Lymphangioma circumscriptum is a microcystic lymphatic malformation characterized by clusters of vesicles that may be clear, yellow, or blood filled. The lesion may have an associated verrucous texture. A common concern for patients with lymphangioma circumscriptum is persistent drainage; CO_2 and Er:YAG lasers can be implemented in an attempt to scar the superficial component and minimize drainage. There have also been reports of successful treatment with PDL for superficial lymphangioma circumscriptum, though the depth of penetration and chromophore target is limited.

Rosacea and telangiectasias

Telangiectasias are small superficial vessels 0.1–1 mm in diameter that are most commonly associated with sun damage or rosacea. There are many other causes of telangiectasias including, though not limited to, connective tissue disease, a host of genodermatoses, and hereditary hemorrhagic telangiectasia. Patients with rosacea often have associated background facial erythema. Lasers and IPL are the treatment of choice for telangiectasias and facial erythema. Flushing can be improved in many patients although recurrence may occur. The most commonly used devices include PDL, KTP, and IPL. Near infra-red lasers, specifically diode and Nd:YAG, have been used to treat deeper or larger-caliber vessels. Treatment must be tailored, taking into account vessel caliber, skin type, and a patient's ability to tolerate purpura.

Typically 3–4 monthly non-purpuric laser treatment sessions with PDL produce a significant reduction in erythema and telangiectasias. (Fig. 2.6) Typical settings include 7–10 mm spot, 6 ms pulse duration, 6–9 J/cm² with epidermal cooling. Lower energies are used with larger spot sizes. Lower fluences should be used for patients with intense facial erythema. Lower fluences and longer pulse durations are advisable in darker skin types. Parameters vary by device. Residual telangiectasias can then be treated with purpuric or non-purpuric settings. Pulse durations of 6 ms and above are typically non-purpuric. Pulse durations of 1.5 ms and 3 ms are likely to induce purpura. Telangiectasia may respond in fewer treatment sessions, and purpuric treatments may be more effective. The end point for treating vessels is vessel clearance, a transient blue coagulum (Video 1), or purpura.

Vessels around the nasal ala can be more challenging to treat, and greater efficacy may be achieved with judicious stacking of non-purpuric PDL pulses. Larger caliber vessels on the nose may require even longer pulse durations and higher fluences. A recent study of 18 patients with

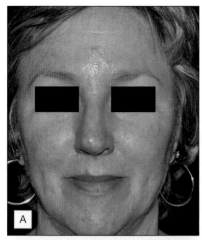

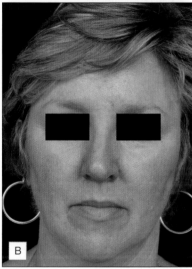

Figure 2.6 Rosacea: (**A**) pre and (**B**) post four pulsed dye laser treatments.

PDL/KTP laser resistant nasal telangiectasia treated with a newer generation PDL utilizing a 40 ms pulse duration and 3 mm × 10 mm elliptical spot showed complete clearance in 10 patients, and >80% improvement in 8 patients.

Background erythema may be treated before or after treating telangiectasias. A cold pack can be applied post-treatment to minimize swelling. Sleeping with several pillows to keep the head elevated can also be helpful if swelling occurs. Rosacea patients should be advised that treatment will significantly reduce erythema and telangiectasias, though maintenance treatments are to be expected as laser is an effective treatment, not a cure.

IPL is also beneficial for the treatment of facial erythema and telangiectasias. The KTP laser may be used to trace individual vessels, with the advantage of no purpura. There is relatively stronger absorption of hemoglobin at 532 nm and care must be taken in patients with darker

skin types. The Nd:YAG laser may also be used to treat refractory nasal vessels and facial reticular veins, though the risk of scarring is increased.

Other vascular lesions

Poikiloderma of Civatte

Poikiloderma of Civatte presents in chronically sun-exposed areas, most commonly on the neck, chest, and lateral cheeks, with red-brown discoloration and associated telangiectasias. IPL may be used for treatment, and has the benefits of targeting both pigmentary and vascular components, as well as availability of larger spot sizes to treat greater surface areas. A report of 175 patients treated with IPL showed clearance of >80% with transient side effects in 5% of patients. Scarring or permanent pigmentary change was not observed. PDL has also been implemented to treat the vascular component of poikiloderma of Civatte with good results. Large spot sizes and relatively lower fluences are advised for PDL to limit potential side effects, most commonly a reticulated pattern and hypopigmentation.

Cherry angiomas

Cherry angiomas are the most common vascular growths of the skin. Cherry angiomas are benign proliferations that tend to be highly responsive to laser treatment. The PDL is commonly used to treat angiomas. The end point is purpura (**Fig. 2.7**). Clearance often occurs with one treatment although there are resistant lesions and larger lesions may require multiple treatments. The KTP laser or IPL may also be utilized.

For larger and thicker angiomas, an initial pulse can be delivered while performing diascopy (compression with a glass slide) to treat the deeper component. After time for cooling, a second pulse may be placed to treat the more superficial component (if the lesion has not become purpuric). Spider angiomas are treated in a similar manner.

Suggested settings with the PDL are 5–7 mm spot, 1.5 ms pulse duration, 7–10 J/cm², with appropriate epidermal cooling. Settings may need to be adjusted for patients with darker skin types. Parameters vary by device. Cherry angiomas may also be treated with electrodesiccation and shave excision.

Venous lakes

Venous lakes are acquired vascular malformations that consist of ectatic venules in the superficial dermis. Venous lakes appear clinically as compressible violaceous papules, and are most commonly located on the lip. Treatment may be initiated for cosmetic purposes or may be prompted by bleeding.

Laser treatment options include PDL for more superficial lesions. For deeper lesions, the diode laser achieves

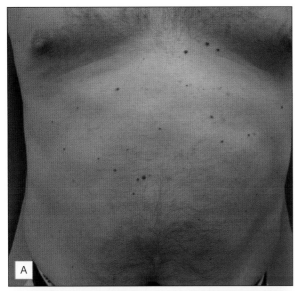

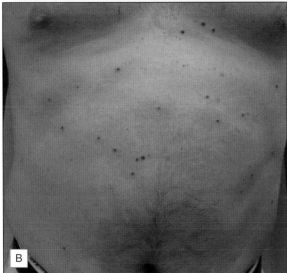

Figure 2.7 Cherry angiomas: (**A**) pre and (**B**) immediately post pulsed dye laser with expected purpura.

Angiokeratomas

Angiokeratomas are characterized by ectatic superficial dermal vessels and overlying hyperkeratosis. Subtypes include solitary or multiple angiokeratomas, which often occur on the lower extremities; angiokeratoma of Fordyce affecting the genital region; angiokeratoma of Mibelli, an autosomal dominant condition typically affecting the dorsal surface of the hands and feet; and angiokeratoma circumscriptum. Angiokeratomas may also be seen in association with Fabry disease, an X-linked recessive disorder characterized by a deficiency of alpha-galactosidase A.

Treatment with vascular specific lasers such as PDL may be initiated to treat the vascular component, though a residual keratotic component may persist. Ablative lasers such as the CO_2 or erbium laser may also be implemented. Scarring can occur with aggressive treatment and in sensitive body areas.

Approach to treatment of vascular lesions

A pre-treatment consultation is advisable, to include a discussion of the amount of improvement expected, number of treatments, expected treatment effects such as erythema, purpura, and swelling, potential adverse effects, and aftercare required (including sun protection and avoidance of trauma). Photos before each treatment are recommended.

Eye protection is essential during treatment. If the treatment area is on the face but outside the orbital rim, metal goggles should be placed over the patient's eyes. Stick-on laser shields with appropriate wavelength protection are useful but careful adherence to the skin is important. An alternative to protect infants and young children's eyes is multiple layers of gauze and a firm gloved hand. Pressure should not be placed on the eye itself, but on the orbital rim. Care must be taken with this approach so that movement of the patient does not expose the eyes. If the treatment area is within the orbital rim, metal eyeshields that are placed under the eyelids and over the cornea must be used. These should be placed with care to avoid corneal abrasions.

Pearl 6

Proper eye protection is essential. Place a corneal metal eyeshield if treatment will be done within the orbital rim.

Many vascular lesion treatments can be done without anesthesia, for example patients with rosacea and telangiectasias. Topical anesthetics can cause blanching of the skin, theoretically decreasing treatment efficacy. Vascular anomalies may be treated with or without anesthesia, taking into account the patient's age, extent of lesion, and preference. Deeper lesions such as venous malformations, or more extensive lesions, may require intralesional lidocaine or nerve blocks. For local infiltration, lidocaine

deeper penetration and is more effective. Alexandrite or Nd:YAG lasers may also be used.

A report by Wall et al suggested the following parameters with a contact cooling diode 800 nm device (Lightsheer ET, Lumenis, Santa Clara, CA): 9 mm spot, 30 ms pulse duration, 40 J/cm², 1–2 pulses. Sapphire chill tip is held on the skin for 2–3 seconds prior to the laser pulse. The end point is flattening, subtle graying, and/or deepening of violaceous color. Suggested PDL settings are 5 or 7 mm spot, 7–10 J/cm², 1.5–6 ms, with appropriate epidermal cooling (e.g. cryogen spray cooling of 30 ms with a 30 ms delay). Settings may need to be adjusted for patients with darker skin types. Parameters vary by device.

without epinephrine is generally used to minimize vasoconstriction.

The approach to treating infants and young children with regards to anesthesia varies widely. There is evidence that early treatment of PWS improves treatment outcome. Treatment without anesthesia in young children may be appropriate for a limited number of pulses. Topical anesthesia can be beneficial, though its use in infants and small children is limited so as not to exceed the maximum recommended dose per package inserts and, as noted above, vasoconstriction can occur. Ulcerated lesions have higher absorption of topical anesthetics and it is advised not to apply topical anesthetics to ulcerated lesions. General anesthesia offers the advantage of avoiding fear and pain in children who will need multiple procedures. It also allows easy placement of the required corneal shield for treatment of eyelid lesions. However, there are risks of general anesthesia. Studies have documented that in healthy patients with vascular lesions the risk is low; however, advantages and disadvantages need to be considered and discussed with the patient and family.

Side effects and complications

The risk from laser treatment of vascular lesions primarily includes scarring and pigmentary changes. The risk of scarring with the PDL is <1%, but is higher for the near-infrared lasers. Scarring can be minimized by performing test pulses and assessing appropriate tissue response before treating the entire lesion. Lasting gray and white discoloration can be signs of necrosis. Pigmentary changes are often transient, although permanent hypopigmentation can occur and can be minimized by avoiding treating tan patients, proper sun protection pre/post treatment, and modifying parameters in darker skin patients. The darker the patient's skin type, the higher is the risk of pigmentary changes. Use of PDL is much more difficult in patients with skin types V and VI. Treatments are less effective owing to melanin blocking light penetration and risk of side effects including pigmentary change and scarring, is higher. In the future, treatments like photodynamic therapy might offer these patients a better treatment option.

Pearl 7

Do not treat tanned skin.

Swelling may also occur with PDL, though is usually mild and transient, resolving within 24–72 hours. Swelling can be more significant when treating vascular malformations with near-infrared lasers that penetrate deeper and with non-purpuric multiple-pass PDL laser technique. More extensive lesions on the lips and tongue may require oral prednisone before treatment to minimize swelling.

Risk of ulceration and scarring is higher with longer wavelength lasers including the alexandrite and Nd:YAG.

Use of these lasers for vascular lesions can require very high energies. These devices should be used cautiously and by clinicians familiar with their use who are prepared to carefully monitor skin effects during and after the procedure. The Nd:YAG in particular has a very narrow therapeutic window.

Further reading

Anderson RR, Parrish JA 1983 Selective photothermolysis: precise microsurgery by selective absorption of pulsed radiation. Science 220:524-527

Bagazgoitia L, Torrelo A, Gutiérrez JC, et al 2011 Propranolol for infantile hemangiomas. Pediatric Dermatology 28:108-114

Batta K, Goodyear HM, Moss C, et al 2002 Randomized controlled study of early PDL treatment of uncomplicated childhood haemangiomas: results of a 1-year analysis. Lancet 360:521-527

Chapas AM, Eickhorst K, Geronemus RG 2007 Efficacy of early treatment of facial port wine stains in newborns: a review of 49 cases. Lasers in Surgery and Medicine 39:563-568

David LR, Malek M, Argenta LC 2003 Efficacy of pulse dye laser therapy for the treatment of ulcerated hemangiomas: a review of 78 patients. British Journal of Plastic Surgery 56:317-327

Finn MC, Glowacki J, Mulliken JB 1983 Congenital vascular lesions: clinical application of a new classification. Journal of Pediatric Surgery 18:894-899

Izikson L, Nelson JS, Anderson RR 2009 Treatment of hypertrophic and resistant port wine stains with a 755 nm laser: a case series of 20 patients. Lasers in Surgery and Medicine 41:427-432

Jia W, Sun V, Tran N, et al 2010 Long-term blood vessel removal with combined laser and topical rapamycin antiangiogenic therapy: implications for effective port wine stain treatment. Lasers in Surgery and Medicine 42:105-112

Madan V, Ferguson F 2010 Using the ultra-long pulse width pulsed dye laser and elliptical spot to treat resistant nasal telangiectasia. Lasers in Medical Science 25:151-154

Maguiness SM, Frieden IJ 2010 Current management of infantile hemangiomas. Seminars in Cutaneous Medicine Surgery 29:106-114

Nguyen CM, Yohn JJ, Weston WL, et al 1998 Facial port wine stains in childhood: prediction of the rate of improvement as a function of age of the patient, size, and location of the port wine stain and the number of treatments with the pulsed dye (585nm) laser. British Journal of Dermatology 138:821-825

Ni N, Langer P, Wagner R, Guo S 2011 Topical timolol for periocular hemangioma: report of further study. Archives of Ophthalmology 129:377-379

Rusciani A, Motta A, Fino P, et al 2008 Treatment of poikiloderma of civatte using intense pulsed light source: 7 years of experience. Dermatologic Surgery 34:314-319

Scherer K, Waner M 2007 Nd:YAG lasers (1,064nm) in the treatment of venous malformations of the face and neck: challenges and benefits. Lasers in Medical Science 22:119-126

Tournas JA, Lai J, Truitt Anne, et al 2009 Combined benzoporphyrin derivative monoacid ring A photodynamic therapy and pulsed dye laser for port wine stain birthmarks. Photodiagnosis and Photodynamic Therapy 6:195-199

Wall TL, Grassi AM, Avram MM 2007 Clearance of multiple venous lakes with an 800-nm diode laser: a novel approach. Dermatologic Surgery 33:100-103

Yang MU, Yaroslavsky AN, Farinelli WA, et al 2005 Long pulsed neodynmium:yttrium-aluminum-garnet laser treatment for port wine stains. Journal of the American Academy of Dermatology 52:480-490

3

Laser treatment of pigmented lesions and tattoos

Kavita Mariwalla, George J. Hruza

Summary and Key Features

- Just as placement of tattoos has gained popularity, so has the number of people interested in their removal

- Black and blue tattoos are the easiest to fade with the most predictable results, whereas multicolored tattoos are the most difficult

- Of the various benign pigmented lesions that can be treated with laser, the easiest to treat are lentigines while the most difficult are the nevi of Ota, Ito, and Hori

- Pigment-specific lasers such as the quality-switched (QS) ruby (694 nm), QS alexandrite (755 nm), and QS Nd:YAG (532 nm and 1064 nm) continue to be the workhorse systems for both tattoo and pigmented lesion removal

- QS lasers remove tattoo pigment through photoacoustic injury, breaking up the ink particles and making them more available for macrophage phagocytosis and removal

- Fractional photothermolysis has provided expanded options for pigmented lesion removal in the last decade, though generally more treatment sessions are required and the cost is higher

- In general, patients with Fitzpatrick skin phototypes I–III have a better response than those with skin phototypes IV–VI as the lasers used for pigment removal can also damage epidermal pigment

- Topical anesthesia is helpful when treating dermal pigmented lesions and tattoos

- Factors to consider prior to estimating the number of treatment sessions a patient will need for tattoo removal include: Fitzpatrick skin phototype, location, color, amount of ink used in the tattoo, scarring or tissue change, and ink layering

- As with any procedure, patient selection and preparation are important to success and photographs of the lesions should be taken prior to each treatment session

- Side effects of laser treatment for pigmented lesions include textural change, scarring, pruritus, hypo- or hyperpigmentation, and immediate pigment change

- Tattoos with white or red ink carry an increased risk of paradoxical darkening after laser treatment, which is why test spots should be carried out prior to the first treatment session

- Caution should be exercised prior to treatment of a tattoo with an allergic reaction as the dispersed ink particles can elicit a systemic response

- For pigmented lesions such as melasma and postinflammatory hyperpigmentation, pre- and postoperative treatment should include hydroquinone and topical retinoids

- Postoperative care includes gentle cleansing and a bland emollient while the skin heals

Introduction

Tattooing has become increasingly popular in recent times, with an estimated 7–20 million people in the USA with at least one. In a 2008 online survey conducted by Harris Interactive, an estimated 14% of all adults in the USA have a tattoo, which corroborates with phone survey results from 2004 in which Laumann & Derick found tattoo prevalence in 26% of males and 22% of females. Interestingly, 17% of those with tattoos considered removal. With advances in laser- and light-based technology, as well as their availability, many patients are not only looking to rid themselves of tattoo ink but also seeking removal of benign pigmented lesions.

In this chapter, we will discuss the use of laser for removing tattoos and ameliorating the appearance of benign pigmented lesions. Although the target for both is pigment, the management of lightening and removal for each condition is distinct.

Pigment removal principles

Quality-switched ('QS') lasers have traditionally been the workhorse laser systems for the removal of pigmentation and tattoos. The laser treatment of pigmented lesions is based on the concept of selective photothermolysis; in essence the chosen laser must emit a wavelength that is specific and well absorbed by the intended target. In the case of tattoos, the chromophore is exogenously placed ink found either within macrophages or extracellularly throughout the dermis. In the case of benign pigmented lesions, the intended chromophore is melanin found within melanocytes, keratinocytes or dermal macrophages. Destruction of this pigment is thought to occur mainly through photoacoustic injury. Because the target particles are small, it is important to use pulses of energy that are extremely short to minimize collateral thermal injury to the normal surrounding tissue. For this reason, QS lasers, with energy pulses in the nanosecond range, enable energy to be deposited very quickly. The intense heat transients cause some particles to shatter and kill the cells in which the pigment resides. The rupture of pigment-containing cells eventually triggers phagocytosis and the packaging of pigment fragments for lymphatic drainage and scavenging by dermal macrophages. For epidermal pigment, the pigment-containing cells are killed with the laser pulses resulting in epidermal necrosis and subsequent sloughing and replacement with normal epidermis.

QS lasers used for pigmented lesions include the QS ruby (694 nm), the QS alexandrite (755 nm) and the QS Nd:YAG (532 and 1064 nm) though it is also possible to use the long-pulsed ruby, alexandrite and diode lasers, or intense pulsed light (see Ch. 5). Within the last decade, fractional photothermolysis ('FP') has gained popularity for its ability to treat pigmented conditions such as melasma, solar lentigines, nevus of Ota, and postinflammatory hyperpigmentation (see Ch. 6).

Lesion selection

Just as important as patient selection is evaluation of the lesion itself. Tattoos can be divided into amateur, professional, cosmetic, medical, and traumatic categories. In amateur tattoos, a steel needle is used to deposit ink, which may be at various depths of the skin, whereas in professional tattoos, a hollow needle is used to inject ink into the dermal layer of skin. Amateur tattoos typically contain pigment of unknown sources such as ash, coal, or India ink (Fig. 3.1). On the other hand, professional tattoo artists often combine ink pigments to achieve novel colors and shading. Cosmetic tattoos using skin-colored tones are important to distinguish, as are medical tattoos such as those used as radiation markers. For traumatic tattoos, it is important to understand the nature of the injury that caused it so as to be aware of the type of material implanted in the skin prior to treatment.

It is critical when treating pigmented lesions other than tattoos that the lesion itself be evaluated for malignancy. Lasers should not be used for any kind of melanoma, as even with in situ melanoma recurrence rates are very high. Similarly, we recommend against the removal of dysplastic nevi with lasers even though studies have shown no

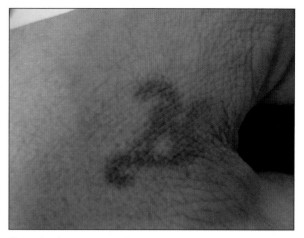

Figure 3.1 Amateur tattoo placed on the hand in a person with Fitzpatrick skin phototype IV.

significant increase in carcinogenic markers after laser stimulation of melanocytes.

Patient selection in general

At initial consultation for removal of a pigmented lesion, it is important to take a thorough medical history including a history of allergy to anesthetics (both topical and injectable), current medical conditions, and medications. If a patient is currently taking isotretinoin, laser treatment should be delayed until medication completion as, theoretically, there is a potential for increased scarring and delayed healing. In addition, it is important to note if the patient was ever treated with systemic gold therapy (e.g. rheumatoid arthritis therapy) as this is an absolute contraindication to QS laser treatment since darkening of gold-containing skin is immediate and irreversible. Prophylaxis is appropriate in patients with a history of herpes simplex virus if treating near the trigger point. A history of keloidal scarring and a tendency toward postinflammatory hypo- or hyperpigmentation should also be documented.

Patient selection for tattoo removal

Though tattoos are increasingly popular, they often become a source of personal regret as up to 50% of adults older than 40 with tattoos seek their removal. It is critical that a thorough history of the tattoo be taken prior to deciding upon a treatment plan to establish appropriate patient expectations (Box 3.1). Kirby et al recently published a scale to help practitioners estimate the number of treatment sessions needed for tattoo removal to appropriately guide patients who often enter the laser removal process of their tattoos with uncertainty and misconceptions (Table 3.1). In the scale, numerical values are assigned to six parameters: (1) Fitzpatrick skin phototype, (2) location, (3) color, (4) amount of ink used in the tattoo, (5) scarring or tissue change, and (6) ink layering. The points for each parameter are combined, which results in the approximate number of treatment sessions needed to successfully remove the tattoo, plus or minus 2.5.

In addition to setting a realistic number of treatment sessions for the patient, it is important to alert the patient that some tattoo pigment may still remain and that hypopigmentation may occur in the area, which will leave the outline of the tattoo sans ink. This is especially true in patients with Fitzpatrick skin phototypes IV–VI or in patients with a tan.

The ideal patient for tattoo removal is an untanned patient with type I or II skin and a dark-blue or black tattoo that has been present for at least a year. The older the tattoo, the better is the response to laser treatment as macrophages are already present in the skin and have been at work trying to actively phagocytose the foreign pigment

particles. This natural attempt by the body to remove the foreign tattoo ink pigment is the reason why older tattoos are often illegible and have blurry or indistinct margins. Multicolored tattoos, regardless of background skin color, can be very difficult to remove completely with traditional laser systems and treatment should be performed only after the patient fully understands the potential for incomplete fading, pigmentary alterations or scarring. Treatment sessions should be spaced at least 6–8 weeks apart.

Patient selection for benign pigmented lesion removal

As with tattoo removal, it is important to assess the patient presenting for benign lesion removal (Box 3.2). The greater the contrast between background skin and pigmented lesion, the more likely the laser surgeon is to achieve success. At preliminary evaluation, a Wood's lamp examination may be helpful to assess depth of pigment. Understanding whether the lesion is epidermal, present at the dermoepidermal junction, or dermal will guide laser selection and also allow the physician to set realistic expectations for removal.

Patients should not be tanned when treated and it is important to stress that regular sunscreen use will aid in a durable result (especially in the case of solar lentigines). In patients with darker skin types, we recommend pretreating pigmented areas with hydroquinone 4% and ceasing treatment 1 week prior to laser therapy. Post-therapy we recommend the use of low potency-topical corticosteroids for 3–4 days to prevent any pigment alteration due to inflammation from the treatment itself. Compared with patients with Fitzpatrick skin phototypes I–III, those with skin photoypes IV–VI have a higher risk of pigmentary alteration and scarring.

Box 3.1
Tattoo lesion patient history

- Is it an amateur, professional, traumatic, cosmetic, or medical tattoo?
- How long has it been present?
- What colors of inks/dyes were used?
- Were inks mixed together to make the colors?
- Is there any white or skin-colored ink in the tattoo to the patient's knowledge?
- Has the patient attempted to remove or alter the tattoo previously? If so, what technique was used?
- Is the patient currently taking a retinoid?
- Is there a history of herpes infection or cold sores in the proposed treatment area?
- Has the patient previously developed keloids or abnormal scars after prior surgery or injury?
- Does the patient currently actively pursue a tan or use a tanning bed or bronzer?
- What is the patient's Fitzpatrick skin type?

Table 3.1 Kirby-Desai scale for estimating number of treatment sessions needed for tattoo removal*

Phototype	Location	Color	Ink amount	Scarring	Layering
I – 1 point	Head and neck – 1 point	Black only – 1 point	Amateur – 1 point	No scar – 0 points	None – 0 points
II – 2 points	Upper trunk – 2 points	Mostly black with some red – 2 points	Minimal – 2 points	Minimal – 1 point	Layering – 2 points
III – 3 points	Lower trunk – 3 points	Mostly black and red with some other colors – 3 points	Moderate – 3 points	Moderate – 3 points	
IV – 4 points	Proximal extremity – 4 points	Multiple colors – 4 points	Significant – 4 points	Significant – 5 points	
V – 5 points	Distal extremity – 5 points				
VI – 6 points					

*Points are listed below each column and assigned depending on six parameters: Fitzpatrick skin phototype, location of the tattoo, color, amount of ink used in the tattoo, scarring and tissue change, and presence or absence of tattoo layering. Physicians should calculate the number using the points listed below each column to arrive at an estimate for number of treatment sessions needed for laser removal (plus or minus 2.5).

Lentigines can be treated most reliably, whereas postinflammatory hyperpigmentation (PIH) and nevi of Ota and Ito present more of a challenge.

Patient preparation

The area to be treated should always be free of any topicals. Removal of pigmented lesions and tattoos can be quite painful for the patient, especially if a large area is to be treated. On the face, we recommend topical anesthetic mixtures that can be compounded at the pharmacy consisting of betacaine, lidocaine, and tetracaine (a typical concentration is 7% of each), or the patient can use a commercial preparation such as LMX-4 or EMLA. A thick layer of this mixture is spread evenly over the treatment area with anesthesia taking place usually within 45 minutes. Penetration of the topical anesthetic can be enhanced by putting the medication under occlusion or applying warm towels over the area. Caution should be exercised if the area is large as topical anesthetics can produce toxicity. Anesthetic should always be completely removed prior to treatment.

Ice is another option, though we recommend ice cubes wrapped in frozen gauze rather than ice packs as the latter tend to not maintain an even temperature. The ice should precede the laser treatment with caution to ensure that no water is left behind. For dermal pigmented lesions on the face, such as nevus of Ota, we sometimes will anesthetize the area with 1% lidocaine.

After informed consent is obtained, pre-treatment photographs are taken. As with any medical procedure, universal precautions should be followed. All QS lasers employ a cone or cylinder placed between the handpiece and the skin to catch any skin debris ejected during laser treatment. Because the cones contain fragments of skin, it is important to use gloves when removing them from the laser after treatment.

Eye safety is also paramount when using lasers. Wavelength-specific protective glasses or goggles must be worn by the patient, provider, and staff at all times during a laser procedure. If the area to be treated is on the eyelid or near the orbit, in the case of the deeply penetrating Nd:YAG 1064 nm laser, internal metal eye shields should be placed for the patient.

Treatment techniques

In general

Prior to commencing full treatment in darkly pigmented individuals, it is advisable to perform test spots on pigmented lesions or tattoos. Test spots should be evaluated at 4–6 weeks for hypo- or hyperpigmentation and efficacy. When using a QS laser, the initial desired response for epidermal and dermoepidermal pigmented lesions is immediate lesion whitening or graying, which represents cavitation. This may be more difficult to gauge if using an IPL system in which the primary endpoint in pigmented lesions is subtle darkening (see Ch. 5). Within 20–30 minutes, this gray converts to erythema. In dermal lesions, the immediate whitening is less vivid.

A snapping sound is common with QS laser use as pigment particles and the cells that contain melanin or tattoo particles are heated and explode. The lesion is fully covered with laser pulses. The immediate whitening keeps additional light from entering the skin due to reflection. Pulse stacking should be avoided as this may increase the risk of scarring and unnecessary thermal injury. If significant energy is absorbed by a pigmented lesion, pinpoint bleeding may occur, as occasionally occurs with tattoos.

Pearl 4

After tattoo treatment, the lesion often turns a gray-white. When treating a multicolored tattoo with more than one laser wavelength, the additional treatment pass should be carried out only after the whitening has fully dissipated, which may take 10–20 minutes.

CASE STUDY 1
Uneven tissue response in a black tattoo

AR is a 39-year-old man with an amateur tattoo on the hand. The tattoo appears black and the patient reports that his 'friend put it there'. The patient does not have a tan. After icing the area for 15 minutes, the tattoo is treated with the QS Nd:YAG laser at a fluence of 3.0 J/cm^2. The tattoo responds immediately and turns white and then erythematous. Unlike the rest of the tattoo, the central portion develops an erosion immediately upon treatment. This occurred because, in amateur tattoos, pigment is not placed at a uniform depth or in a uniform concentration. The tattoo was treated from the periphery to the center. While the periphery responded well, it was too much energy for the center, which led to immediate epidermal sloughing and pinpoint bleeding (Figs 3.1 and 3.2).

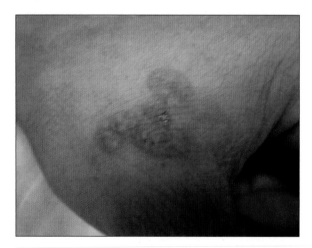

Figure 3.2 Amateur tattoo immediately after treatment with the QS Nd:YAG laser showing punctuate bleeding.

Performing 2–4 treatments of a tattoo all in one day (waiting for the immediate whitening to fade between treatments) seems to increase the degree of fading achieved in one visit.

Patients and equipment for dark-blue or black tattoo treatment

Fitzpatrick skin phototypes I–III

In lighter-skinned patients (in the absence of a tan or bronzer), the practitioner has several options (Table 3.2). The QS alexandrite (755 nm), the QS ruby (694 nm), and the QS Nd:YAG (1064 nm) lasers are all effective for dark-blue and black tattoos (Fig. 3.3). In the case of traumatic tattoos that appear black, it is important to know the origin of the trauma since such tattoos may react with a small explosion (e.g. gun powder tattoo) after laser treatment.

Fitzpatrick skin phototypes IV–VI

In darker-skinned patients, lasers having longer wavelengths are generally safer as they spare the epidermis to a greater degree than shorter-wavelength lasers. Thus, the QS Nd:YAG (1064 nm) is the laser of choice.

Patients and equipment for red tattoo treatment

The optimal laser wavelength for removing red tattoo ink is 532 nm (QS frequency-doubled Nd:YAG). This wavelength can cause both hyperpigmentation and hypopigmentation in darker-skinned patients so treatment should be limited to phototype I–III patients. It should be noted that red tattoo ink is often the culprit for allergic reactions after tattoo placement and granulomatous reactions in the tattoo itself (Fig. 3.4). Laser removal of the red ink can cause greater dispersion of the antigen resulting in urticaria or a systemic allergic reaction. In these cases, an ablative CO$_2$ or Er:YAG laser can be employed to vaporize the tattoo (Fig. 3.5). If a QS-laser is employed, the patient should be covered with systemic corticosteroids and antihistamines and the laser surgeon should proceed with caution (Case study 2).

Table 3.2 Laser choices based on tattoo ink color

QS laser	Black	Blue	Green	Red
Alexandrite 755 nm	X	X	X	
Ruby 694 nm	X	X	X	
Nd:YAG 1064 nm	X	X	X	
Nd:YAG 532 nm				X
Nd:YAG 650 nm			X	

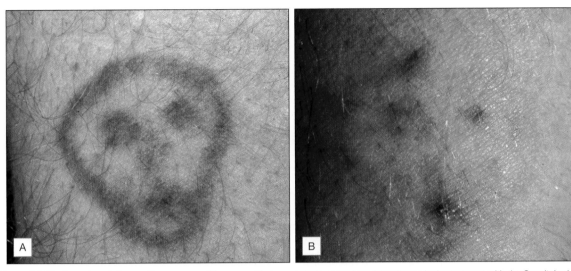

Figure 3.3 Black amateur tattoo on the arm seen (**A**) preoperatively, and (**B**) 6 weeks later following a single treatment with the Q-switched ruby laser with only small speckles of ink remaining.

CASE STUDY 2
When laser removal is not an option

TV is a 53-year-old woman who decided to have a red daisy on a green stem placed on her ankle 1 year ago. Approximately 3 months after getting the tattoo, she complained of itching in the area and noticed a gradual thickening of the skin. She had not experienced this with her other tattoos and has one on the dorsal foot of the same lower extremity that was normal in appearance. She tried clobetasol cream to the area, which initially helped and then failed and then she used flurandrenolide (Cordran®) tape, which worked to alleviate the itch but not the size of the reaction in the area. On exam, the patient is skin phototype V with a thick plaque on the ankle in which one can begin to make out individual flower petals. No visible red ink remained but the green stem was still present. Given her background skin tone and history of red ink, the decision was made to forgo laser therapy of the area in favor of surgical excision. The pathology showed a pseudolymphoma resulting from a granulomatous reaction to the red ink. In this case, QS laser therapy would have been of minimal benefit and surgical therapy became the mainstay of treatment (Fig. 3.6).

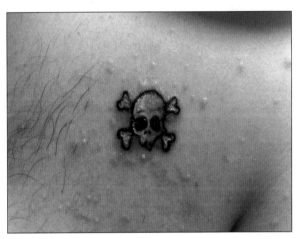

Figure 3.4 Multicolored tattoo showed allergy to yellow ink. The area was successfully treated with Class I topical corticosteroids thus avoiding the need to remove the tattoos with laser.

Patients and equipment for epidermal lesions
Solar lentigines, lentigo simplex, and ephelides

Pigment that is in the epidermis accounts for lesions such as solar lentigines, lentigo simplex, and ephelides. Any laser system that damages the epidermis will therefore result in improvement in 1–2 treatment sessions (Fig. 3.7). Conversely, if the epidermal damage is part of a deeper destruction, there may be scarring or dyspigmentation afterward. Fractional photothermolysis can be considered for these conditions especially if the lesions are widespread (see Ch. 6), but the mainstay lasers are the QS alexandrite, QS Nd:YAG (532 nm), and QS ruby lasers. Long-pulsed lasers and IPL can also be effective (see Ch. 5).

Patients and equipment for green tattoo treatment

The optimal laser wavelength for removing green tattoo ink is the QS ruby laser (694 nm). Because this wavelength is well absorbed by melanin, caution should be used, as injury to melanocytes can lead to transient hypopigmentation and even permanent depigmentation as well as textural change. The goal of treatment should be immediate tissue whitening with minimal or no bleeding.

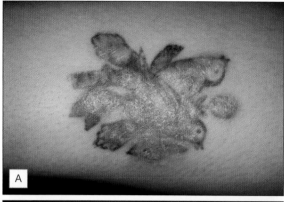

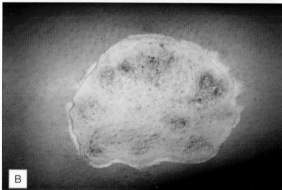

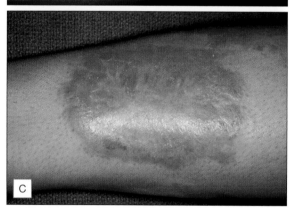

Figure 3.5 Tattoo granulomas from an allergic reaction to the red (cinnabar or mercury tattoo ink) color in a multicolored tattoo seen (**A**) preoperatively, (**B**) immediately after removal of the tattoo and all granulomas with the vaporizational mode of the carbon dioxide laser, and (**C**) 3 months later showing the residual erythematous permanent scar.

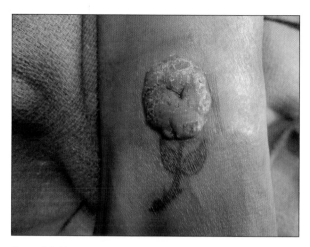

Figure 3.6 Biopsy proven pseudolymphoma in the portions of the tattoo decorated with red ink.

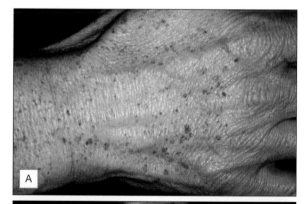

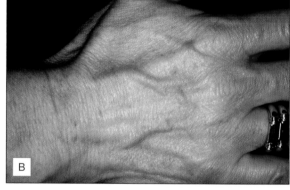

Figure 3.7 Multiple small brown lentigines on the back of the hand seen (**A**) preoperatively, and (**B**) with nearly complete resolution 6 weeks after a single treatment with the Q-switched Nd:YAG laser.

Labial melanotic macules

Melanotic macules on the lip vermilion are a feature of several entities including physiological racial pigmentation, Laugier-Hunziker syndrome, and Peutz-Jeghers syndrome. These can be treated using the QS ruby or QS alexandrite or frequency-doubled QS Nd:YAG lasers. In the case of the syndromes, patients should be made aware that new macules will develop over time (Fig. 3.8).

Café au lait macules and nevus spilus

Café-au-lait macules ('CALM') vary in color, size, and shape but histologically the excess pigment is found at the basal layer. When darker macules exist with the CALM, it is referred to as a nevus spilus. Before treating CALMS, one should always take a careful history to rule out neurofibromatosis (if multiple macules exist). Lasers that are usually used to treat these lesions include the QS Nd:YAG, QS ruby, and QS alexandrite lasers. Patients with darker skin are at risk for hyperpigmentation and hypopigmentation. Light-skinned patients are the ideal candidates for CALM removal, but recurrences, residual hyperpigmentation, and incomplete pigment removal are common. Treatment sessions are spaced at least 8 weeks apart and clearance requires at least 2–4 treatment sessions (Fig. 3.9).

Patients and equipment for dermoepidermal lesions

Lesions in this category include Becker's nevus, melasma, postinflammatory hyperpigmentation, drug-induced

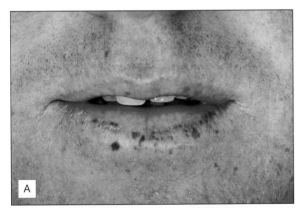

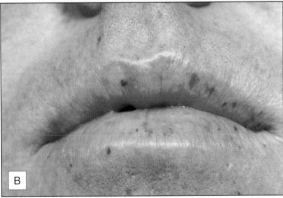

Figure 3.8 Multiple small lentigines of the oral mucosa seen with Peutz-Jeghers syndrome seen (**A**) preoperatively, and (**B**) 6 weeks after three treatments with the Q-switched ruby laser showing excellent fading without scarring.

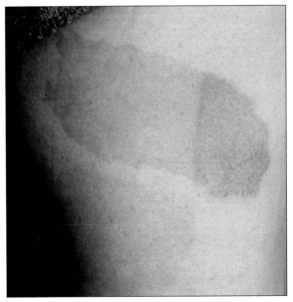

Figure 3.9 Solitary café au lait patch on the leg showing the complication of hyperpigmentation of the lateral portion of the lesion 12 weeks after testing with the Q-switched Nd:YAG laser.

hyperpigmentation, and nevocellular nevi. Pigment is present at the dermoepidermal junction and, in the case of a Becker's nevus, in addition to the pigment there are often terminal hairs in the lesion itself. Nevocellular, junctional, and compound melanocytic nevi should be treated with laser only if the operator is certain that they are benign.

Becker's nevus

The hyperpigmented areas of a Becker's nevus have shown improvement when treated with the QS ruby, QS Nd:YAG, and 1550 nm fractional erbium-doped fiber laser. Of the QS lasers, the ruby is slightly more effective than the Nd:YAG. Treatment sessions should be spaced 8–12 weeks apart and 3–5 treatment sessions are usually necessary. With any of these methods, fading is generally incomplete and patchy. The terminal hairs can be removed with hair removal lasers (see Ch. 4).

Melasma

Melasma is caused by a number of factors including hormonal changes, sun exposure, and medication use. It typically presents as patchy hyperpigmented areas on the face in women. Unfortunately, although lasers can improve the appearance of melasma, this is usually short-lived as recurrences are common. Patients must be counseled on the proper use of broad-spectrum sunscreen at all times and be aware that treatment of melasma may result in postinflammatory hyperpigmentation ('PIH'). The QS ruby, QS alexandrite, QS Nd:YAG, Er:YAG, 1550 nm fractionated erbium doped fiber laser, and fractional CO_2 laser have all been reported as treatment modalities to improve melasma although there is no definitive cure. Worsening of the melasma and recurrence after 'successful' treatment are frequently seen. Treatment sessions are usually spaced 4–8 weeks apart and 4–8 sessions are needed. It is important to not attempt correction of melasma during spring or summer as incidental sunlight exposure will likely counteract any improvement made by the laser itself. As with PIH, pre-treatment with topical hydroquinone or with Kligman's formula (5% hydroquinone, 0.1% tretinoin, 0.1% dexamethasone) is likely to enhance results and these topicals should be continued as part of a maintenance regimen.

Postinflammatory hyperpigmentation

PIH occurs due to hemosiderin and/or melanin deposition. Because this condition arises due to inflammation, it is important to use low fluences and ensure that the patient does not develop significant post-treatment erythema to provoke additional PIH. For this reason, test spots are encouraged prior to treating large areas. The laser system currently used most often for PIH is the fractional photothermolysis system, even though treatment with this laser has been reported to induce PIH itself (see Ch. 6). PIH can occur on the face, but can also be a result of hemosiderin deposition after sclerotherapy. For post-sclerotherapy hyperpigmentation, the QS ruby or IPL (see

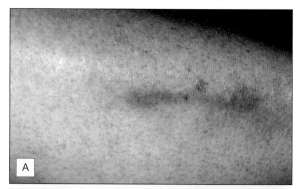

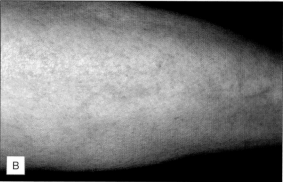

Figure 3.10 Area of postinflammatory hyperpigmentation following sclerotherapy for small leg veins seen (**A**) preoperatively, and (**B**) 6 weeks after multiple treatments with the Q-switched ruby laser.

Ch. 5) can be used (Fig. 3.10). All patients being treated for PIH on the face should use topical hydroquinone 4% cream along with a broad-spectrum sunscreen before and after treatment. Before using a laser for facial PIH, we recommend a trial of topical retinoids and a series of chemical peels to try to improve the discoloration with laser as the final step. Recurrence is frequently seen, especially after sun exposure.

Pearl 7

Controversy exists regarding the long-term use of hydroquinone. Although it is reasonable to offer patients peels, there are over-the-counter preparations that are hydroquinone free if the patient wishes to maintain their post-laser results. Ingredients in these hydroquinone-free products include compounds such as kojic acid, anisic acid, and arbutin.

Drug-induced hyperpigmentation

Minocycline, doxycycline, amiodarone, and azidothymidine (AZT, zidovudine) can cause hyperpigmentation of the skin that appears as gray-brown to brown. Type II minocycline hyperpigmentation has been reported to clear after use of the QS alexandrite laser and the QS Nd:AG laser. Discontinuation of the medication is important and treatments should be started after a trial of hydroquinone 4%.

Congenital nevi

Congenital nevi that are too large for surgical removal may be considered for treatment with laser. Unfortunately, scarring is common especially on the anterior torso, flanks, or arms. Authors have reported success with the QS lasers in the past, and more recently the Er : YAG and the CO_2, or a combination of the QS lasers with ablative resurfacing. It is important to note that most studies have evaluated children with congenital nevi rather than adults who desire removal and, in general, the value of removing congenital nevi with any laser has not been substantiated as residual pigment and repigmentation are common.

Patients and equipment for dermal lesions

Dermal lesions have pigment deeper in the dermis that require devices with longer wavelengths. Examples of such lesions include nevi of Ota, Ito, and Hori, and congenital dermal melanocytosis also known as Mongolian spots. Argyria is an additional example of a dermal process that manifests as a result of ingestion of silver and can be treated with QS laser.

Nevi of Ota, Ito, and Hori

Nevus of Ota presents on the face as a blue-black, brown, or gray patch that develops after birth or in adolescence with a unilateral distribution that may involve the sclera. Nevus of Ito is similar, but its location is usually on the shoulder. Hori's nevus is typically bilateral and located in the malar region. In darker-skinned (type IV–VI) patients, the QS Nd : YAG laser at 1064 nm is usually the safest laser to lighten a nevus of Ota, Ito or Hori. In lighter-skinned patients, QS ruby laser at 694 nm and QS alexandrite laser at 755 nm can also be used (Fig. 3.11). Recently, a fractionated 1440 nm Nd : YAG laser has been reported to clear nevus of Ota. Treatments are usually spaced 3–4 months apart with up to 10 treatment sessions needed for clearance with QS lasers, and 2–3 treatment sessions with the fractionated laser. Nevus of Ota patients should be made aware that the sclera component of the lesion is not amenable to treatment with current technology.

Congenital dermal melanocytosis

Mongolian spots typically appear as blue-gray macules of varying size on the body that resolve in childhood but occasionally persist into adulthood. These can be treated with the QS alexandrite, ruby or Nd : YAG laser though PIH is a risk. Sacral spots tend to be more laser-resistant than extrasacral Mongolian spots and treatment in childhood portends better results.

Argyria

Argyria is a rare skin disease caused by ingestion of silver salt or silver particles used in traditional remedies. The

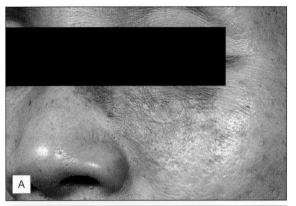
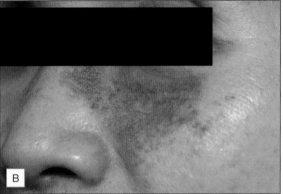
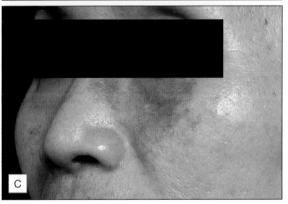

Figure 3.11 Small nevus of Ota is seen: (**A**) preoperatively, (**B**) 6 weeks after two treatments with the Q-switched ruby laser showing some fading, and (**C**) with nearly complete fading 6 weeks after the fourth treatment.

pigment granules that result in the blue-gray discoloration associated with argyria are usually found in the upper dermis. Treatment of argyria can be successfully accomplished using the QS 1064 nm Nd : YAG at low fluences. Special attention should be given to anesthesia in this situation as treatment is very painful.

Amalgam tattoos

Amalgam tattoos on the gingival or buccal mucosa result from placement of silver fillings in the teeth and can be of cosmetic concern especially if on the anterior gingival surface. These metallic deposits can be removed using the QS ruby or QS alexandrite laser.

Pearl 8

In order to anesthetize the gingiva, consider tetracaine gel. Application is done with a cotton tip applicator and onset of action is usually under 1 minute. It is important, however, that the gel be removed with gauze prior to laser treatment.

Postoperative care

If a Q-switched laser was used for treatment of dermal lesions, the area will appear somewhat abraded after treatment. Apply a layer of petrolatum beneath a dressing of non-stick gauze and paper tape. Instruct the patient to change the dressing daily after first gently cleansing the area with soap and water. This should be continued until the area has completely re-epithelialized. A dry crust should never be allowed to form. The treatment area should heal within 5–14 days. No specific wound care is needed after the treatment of epidermal lesions. A very subtle eschar appearing as a darker version of the original lesion will form and peel off within 7–10 days.

If an IPL system was used for treatment, typically only erythema is seen postoperatively and dressings are not generally required (see Ch. 5). After fractional photothermolysis, broad-spectrum sunscreen and non-comedogenic moisturizer should be applied for at least 1 week (see Ch. 6).

Troubleshooting for tattoo removal

When evaluating a tattoo patient prior to initiating therapy, carefully palpate and examine the site to be sure that no pre-existing scarring, hypopigmentation, or induration is present. Many patients may not realize that the actual tattooing procedure can cause both scars and loss of normal pigmentation.

Incomplete removal of the tattoo is a common problem following laser treatment. If treatment is ineffective, an increase in energy fluence may be necessary, but care must always be taken to stay within safe treatment parameters to avoid scarring or pigmentary alterations. In some cases, changing to a different laser may be worthwhile due to the intrinsic differences in wavelengths, pulse durations, and spot sizes.

Troubleshooting for pigmented lesion removal

As with tattoos, incomplete removal of benign pigmented lesions following laser treatment is the chief problem. However, unlike tattoos, only a few additional treatments will usually lead to total or near-total removal of CALMs, lentigines, and nevi of Ota and Ito. Increasing the energy fluence often produces improvement in resistant lesions.

When treating lentigines, if the patient has lesions on both their hands and face, it is always best to treat the hand lesions first so that if an untoward reaction results it will result in less patient unhappiness than if the same problem had developed on the face. This is especially true in patients with darker skin types. However, the face heals much faster and tends to be more forgiving than the hands.

Side effects and complications

Alterations in pigmentation

Despite appropriate precautions, pigmentary alteration can still occur following laser treatment of tattoos or benign pigmented lesions. The hyperpigmentation usually improves with time or use of topical bleaching creams such as 4–5% hydroquinone compounded with 1–2% hydrocortisone and 0.0–0.1% tretinoin. Hypopigmentation is more difficult to treat, but the use of the excimer laser or narrow band ultraviolet (UVB) light may help. Still, multiple treatments are often required and incomplete resolution is common. Whereas many cases of pigmentary alteration will resolve spontaneously over time, some cases may be permanent.

If a patient who has taken gold therapy is inadvertently treated with a QS laser, immediate darkening of the gold particles in the skin may result. This is thought to occur due to alteration in the gold particles present in the skin. A long-pulsed ruby laser has been reported to clear the resultant discoloration.

In skin phototypes IV–VI, decorative tattoo removal can be especially challenging as the current devices used to treat tattoos are also used to treat benign pigmented lesions. As a consequence, complications such as epidermal blistering, hypopigmentation, and incomplete tattoo removal can be anticipated and should be evaluated through test spots prior to the first treatment session. Waiting 6–8 weeks prior to full treatment will allow such pigmentary complications to reveal themselves so the laser surgeon can plan appropriately.

Pearl 9

If a test spot darkens on a cosmetic facial tattoo, rather than try to treat the dark spot, consider surgical excision of the test spot and proceeding with ablative and/or fractional resurfacing.

Paradoxical darkening of tattoo pigment

Cosmetic tattooing is the process of using tattoo ink to enhance the shape of the lips, to augment the appearance of the eyebrow, to accentuate eyelids, or to reconstruct the appearance of the areola following mastectomy. When a patient desires subsequent removal of this type of tattoo, extreme caution should be exercised, because in most of these situations white ink pigment has been used to achieve the skin-colored tattoo tone. In non-cosmetic tattoos, the presence of pastel colors such as light blue, turquoise, yellow, light green, lavender, and pink should also raise suspicion of white ink additives. Treatment may result in immediate and permanent tattoo darkening in white and even in red tattoos. The laser pulse can reduce ink from rust-colored ferric oxide (Fe_2O_3) to jet-black ferrous oxide (FeO). Similarly, white ink made up of titanium dioxide (TiO_2, T^{4+}) can be reduced to blue Ti^{3+} upon laser treatment. Such post-treatment darkening appears immediately. For this reason, a single small inconspicuous test spot is recommended to ensure that this complication does not occur. Even after testing, it is appropriate to obtain the patient's written consent that they understand tattoo ink darkening may still occur during future treatments and that it may be permanent. The darkening usually becomes apparent once the immediate whitening has faded. If pigment darkening does occur in a decorative tattoo, it may be improved with subsequent treatment with the QS Nd:YAG laser operated at 1064 nm.

Thermal injury and scarring

Textural changes can be minimized through use of a large spot size and appropriate spacing of treatments at 6–8 weeks. Significant thermal injury and subsequent scarring are rare (~5%) when treating dermal pigmented lesions if the proper laser guidelines are followed and the appropriate treatment parameters are used. When they do occur, they are most likely to happen on the chest, outer upper arm and ankle. Ideal wound care with normal saline cleansing and application of petrolatum with a non-stick gauze dressing may prevent infection and help to minimize scarring. In spite of these efforts, if scarring does occur, subsequent treatment with a series of pulsed dye laser treatments, a series of injections of low-dose triamcinolone acetonide directly into the scar or topical application of silicone gel sheeting along with scar massage over a period of several weeks may help to improve the appearance of the scar. Cobblestone texture seen within 2 weeks of treatment is a sign of incipient scarring, and may be reversed with twice daily application of class I topical corticosteroids. Scarring after QS laser treatment of epidermal lesions is extremely rare.

Special situations

Tattoo granulomas

Allergic granulomas to tattoo ink are probably most commonly seen to the cinnabar in red-colored inks. In these situations, the use of any of the QS lasers is not recommended as it may worsen the allergic reaction and produce systemic symptoms or even anaphylactic reactions. The use of an ablative laser, such as the carbon dioxide or Er:YAG laser, can be employed to remove the offending ink and also destroy the granulomas at the same time. Biopsies should be considered before laser treatment to rule out sarcoidosis, infectious granulomas such as atypical mycobacterial infections, and other entities.

Table 3.3 Tattoo pigments used to create specific tattoo colors

Tattoo color	Source
Black	Carbon, iron oxide, India ink, lead, gunpowder
Red	Cinnabar (mercuric sulfide), cadmium selenide, sienna, azo dyes
Green	Chromium oxide, malachite green, hydrated chromium sesquioxide, lead chromate
Blue	Cobalt aluminum
Brown	Ochre
Yellow	Cadmium sulfide, ochre, curcumin yellow
Violet	Manganese violet
White	Titanium dioxide, zinc oxide

Multicolored tattoos

When treating a tattoo of multiple colors, especially black, red, or green, more than one laser may be required to maximize the degree of improvement. In these situations, the black outline of the tattoo is usually first treated with infrared light from the QS Nd:YAG laser operated at 1064 nm. Once that portion of the treatment has been completed, the green light from the frequency-doubled QS Nd:YAG laser operated at 532 nm is used to treat the red portions of the tattoo. If green tattoo ink is also present, red light from the Q-switched ruby or alexandrite lasers is used. Alternatively, the QS Nd:YAG with a 650 nm wavelength dye-containing handpiece can be used as well. Care should be taken to avoid overlapping the treatment pulses as much as possible by matching the size of the laser beam to the amount of the tattoo color being treated. By using this technique, it is often possible to treat the entire tattoo at one time resulting in more rapid resolution of the different colors than if they were treated individually at different visits. Other colors respond unpredictably to specific wavelengths with the treatment done mostly by trial and error. If prominent immediate whitening in the tattoo ink is noted, that laser wavelength will tend to achieve fading of that color (Table 3.3).

Further reading

Adrian RM, Griffin L 2000 Laser tattoo removal. Clinics in Plastic Surgery 27:181-192

Anderson RR, Geronemus R, Kilmer SL, et al 1993 Cosmetic tattoo ink darkening. A complication of Q-switched and pulsed-laser treatment. Archives of Dermatology 129(8): 1010-1014

Anderson RR, Parrish JA 1983 Selective photothermolysis: precise microsurgery by selective absorption of pulsed radiation. Science 220(4596):524-527

Armstrong ML, Roberts AE, Koch JR et al 2008 Motivation for contemporary tattoo removal a shift in identity. Archives of Dermatology 144:879-884

Ashinoff R, Levine VJ, Soter NA 1995 Allergic reactions to tattoo pigment after laser treatment. Dermatologic Surgery 21(4):291-294

Choi JE, Kim JW, Seo SH, et al 2009 Treatment of Becker's nevi with a long-pulsed alexandrite laser. Dermatologic Surgery 35:1105-1108

Duke D, Byers HR, Sober AJ 1999 Treatment of benign and atypical nevi with the normal-mode ruby laser and the Q-switched ruby laser: clinical improvement but failure to completely eliminate nevomelanocytes. Archives of Dermatology 135:290-296

Fitzpatrick RE, Goldman MP 1994 Tattoo removal using the alexandrite laser. Archives of Dermatology 130(12):1508-1514

Grevelink JM, Duke D, van Leeuwen RL, et al 1996 Laser treatment of tattoos in darkly pigmented patients: efficacy and side effects. Journal of the American Academy of Dermatology 34:653-656

Hantash BM, Bedi VP, Sudireddy V, et al 2006 Laser-induced transepidermal elimination of dermal content by fractional photothermolysis. Journal of Biomedical Optics 11:041115

Jeong SY, Shin JB, Yeo UC, et al 2010 Low-fluence Q switched neodymium-doped yttrium aluminum garnet laser for melasma with pre- or post-treatment triple combination cream. Dermatologic Surgery 36:1-10

Kagami S, Asahina A, Watanabe R, et al 2008 Laser treatment of 26 Japanese patients with Mongolian spots. Dermatologic Surgery 34:1689-1694

Katz TM, Goldberg LH, Firoz BF, et al 2009 Fractional photothermolysis for the treatment of postinflammatory hyperpigmentation. Dermatologic Surgery 35: 1844-1948

Kilmer SL, Anderson RR 1993 Clinical use of the Q-switched ruby and the Q-switched Nd:YAG (1064 nm and 532 nm) lasers for treatment of tattoos. Journal of Dermatologic Surgery and Oncology 19(4):330-338

Kilmer SL 2002 Laser eradication of pigmented lesions and tattoos. Dermatologic Clinics 20:37-53

Kirby W, Desai A, Desai T, et al 2009 The Kirby-Desai scale: a proposed scale to assess tattoo-removal treatments. Journal of Clinical and Aesthetic Dermatology 2(3): 32-37

Kono T, Nozaki M, Chan HH, et al 2001 A retrospective study looking at the long-term complications of Q-switched ruby laser in the treatment of nevus of Ota. Lasers in Surgery and Medicine 29:156-159

Laubach H, Tannous Z, Anderson RR, et al 2006 Skin responses to fractional photothermolysis. Lasers in Surgery and Medicine 38:142-149

Laumann AE, Derick AJ 2006 Tattoos and body piercings in the United States: a national data set. Journal of the American Academy of Dermatology 55:413-421

Polder KD, Landau JM, Vergilis-Kalner IJ, et al 2011 Laser eradication of pigmented lesions: a review. Dermatologic Surgery 37:572-595

Laser hair removal

Omar A. Ibrahimi, Suzanne L. Kilmer

4

Summary and Key Features

- Laser hair removal is the most commonly requested cosmetic procedure in the world

- The extended theory of selective photothermolysis enables the laser surgeon to target and destroy hair follicles, thereby leading to both permanent and temporary hair removal

- The ideal candidate for laser hair removal (LHR) is fair skinned with dark terminal hair; however, LHR can today be successfully performed in all skin types

- Thin hairs and hairs with white, blond and red color are extremely difficult to treat with laser hair removal devices

- Wax epilation should be avoided prior to laser hair removal treatments

- Lasers pose a safety risk to both the patient and device operator

- Informed consent should be reviewed with every patient prior to treatment

- Wavelengths, spot size, pulse duration, and skin cooling are key variables that can be used to tailor laser–tissue interactions for a given patient

- Roughly 15–30% of hairs can be removed with each treatment session using ideal parameters. Remaining hairs are often thinner and lighter in color

- The most common complication is pigmentary alteration, which can be temporary or permanent

Introduction

The non-specific damage of human hair follicles with a laser was noted over 50 years ago. However, it was not until the theory of selective photothermolysis was proposed by two Harvard dermatologists, Rox Anderson and John Parrish, that the concept of selectively targeting a particular chromophore based on its absorption spectra and size was realized. In 1996, this group also reported the first successful use of a normal-mode ruby laser for long-term and permanent hair removal.

Removing unwanted body hair is today a worldwide trend, and hair removal using laser or other light-based technology is one of the most highly requested cosmetic procedures. Prior to the advent of laser hair removal (LHR), only temporary methods for removing unwanted hair were available such as bleaching, plucking, shaving, waxing, and chemical depilatories. Threading, a form of epilation using a cotton thread, is a common practice in some cultures. In addition to not providing permanent hair removal, these methods are also inconvenient and tedious. Electrolysis is a technique in which a fine needle is inserted deep into the hair follicle and uses electrical current, thereby destroying the hair follicle and allowing for permanent hair removal of all types of hair. However, this technique is impractical for treating large areas, extremely tedious, operator dependent, and with variable efficacy in achieving permanent hair removal. Eflornithine (α-difluoromethylornithine or DFMO) is a topical inhibitor of ornithine decarboxylase that slows the rate of hair growth and is currently FDA cleared for the removal of unwanted facial hair in women. In this chapter, we provide a detailed overview on LHR including discussion of hair follicle biology, the science behind LHR, key factors in optimizing treatment, and future trends.

Basic hair biology

The hair follicle is a hormonally active structure (Fig. 4.1) that is anatomically divided into an infundibulum (hair follicle orifice to insertion of the sebaceous gland), isthmus (insertion of the sebaceous gland to the insertion of the arrector (erector) pili muscle), and inferior (insertion of the arrector pili to the base of the hair follicle) segments. The dermal papilla provides neurovascular support to the base of the follicle and helps form the hair shaft.

Every hair follicle is controlled by a programmed cycle that is dependent on the anatomical location. The hair cycle consists of anagen, catagen, and telogen phases. Anagen is characterized by a period of active growth where the hair shaft lengthens. A catagen transition period follows in which the lower part of the hair follicle undergoes apoptosis. A resting period, telogen, then ensues, and regrowth occurs when anagen resumes. Hair regrowth (entry into another anagen cycle) is dependent on stem cells within or near the hair bulb matrix. Slow-cycling stem cells have also been found in the follicular bulge

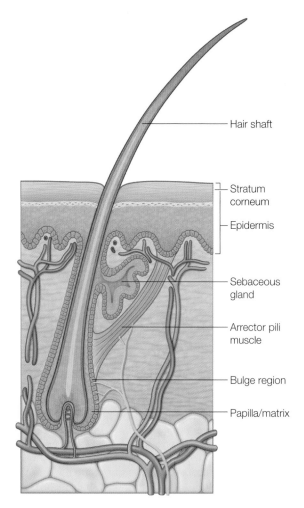

Hair shaft

Stratum corneum

Epidermis

Sebaceous gland

Arrector pili muscle

Bulge region

Papilla/matrix

Figure 4.1 Hair follicle anatomy. *Reproduced from Tsao SS, Hruza GJ 2005 Laser hair removal. In: Robinson JK, Hanke CW, Sengelmann RD, Siegel DM (eds) Surgery of the Skin. Elsevier Mosby, Philadelphia, p 575-588.*

arising off the outer root sheath at the site of the arrector pili muscle attachment.

The main types of hair include lanugo, vellus, and terminal hairs. Lanugo hairs are fine hairs that cover a fetus and are shed in the neonatal period. Vellus hairs are usually non-pigmented, and have a diameter of roughly 30–50 μm. Terminal hair shafts range from 150 to 300 μm in diameter. The type of hair produced by an individual follicle is capable of change (e.g. vellus to terminal hair at puberty or terminal to vellus hair in androgenic alopecia).

The amount and type of pigment in the hair shaft determine hair color. Melanocytes produce two types of melanin: eumelanin, a brown-black pigment; and pheomelanin, a red pigment. Melanocytes are located in the upper portion of the hair bulb and outer root sheath of the infundibulum.

Definitions of what constitutes excessive or unwanted body hair depends on cultural mores, but can usually be classified as either hypertrichosis or hirsutism. Hirsutism is the abnormal growth of terminal hair in women in male-pattern (androgen-dependent) sites such as the face and chest. Hypertrichosis is excess hair growth at any body site that is not androgen dependent. Additionally, the use of grafts and flaps in skin surgery can often introduce hair to an area that causes a displeasing appearance or functional impairment.

Mechanism of LHR

The theory of selective photothermolysis enables precise targeting of pigmented hair follicles by using the melanin of the hair shaft as a chromophore. Melanin has an absorbance spectrum that matches wavelengths in the red and near-infrared (IR) portion of the electromagnetic spectrum. To achieve permanent hair removal, the biological 'target' is the follicular stem cells located in the bulge region and/or dermal papilla. Due to the slight spatial separation of the chromophore and desired target, an extended theory of selective photothermolysis was proposed that requires diffusion of heat from the chromophore to the desired target for destruction. This requires a laser pulse duration that is longer in duration than if the actual chromophore and desired target are identical. Temporary LHR can result when the follicular stem cells are not completely destroyed, primarily through induction of a catagen-like state in pigmented hair follicles. Temporary LHR is much easier to achieve than permanent removal when using lower fluences. Long-term hair removal depends on hair color, skin color, and tolerated fluence. Roughly 15–30% long-term hair loss may be observed with each treatment when optimal treatment parameters are used (Fig. 4.2). A list of laser and light devices that are currently commercially available for hair removal is given in Table 4.1.

Key factors in optimizing treatment

LHR has revolutionized the ability to eliminate unwanted hair temporarily and permanently in many individuals of all skin colors. Proper patient selection, preoperative preparation, informed consent, understanding of the principles of laser safety, and laser and light source selection are key to the success of laser treatment. An understanding of hair anatomy, growth and physiology, together with a thorough understanding of laser–tissue interaction, in particular within the context of choosing optimal laser parameters for effective LHR, should be acquired before using lasers for hair removal.

Patient selection

A focused medical history, physical examination, and informed consent, including setting realistic expectations and potentials risks, should be performed prior to any

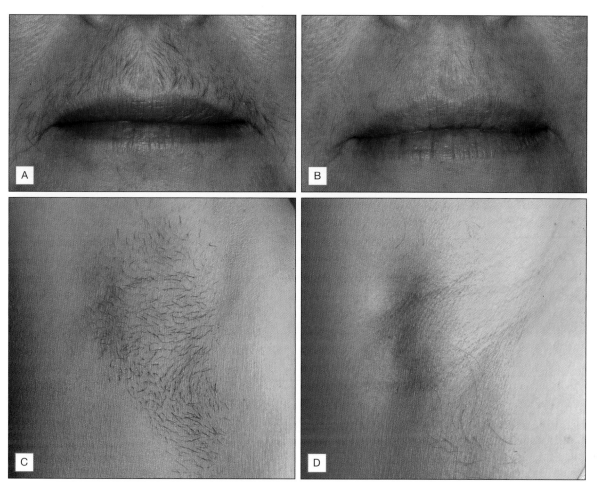

Figure 4.2 Laser hair removal is safe and effective. (**A**) The upper cutaneous lip of a hirsute female. (**B**) Appearance of same subject following only three treatments with a long-pulsed 755 nm alexandrite laser used with a 12 mm spot size, 16 J/cm², 3 ms pulse duration and DCD setting of 30/30/0. (**C**) Axilla of an adult female. (**D**) Following four treatments with a long-pulsed diode laser with a large spot size and vacuum-assisted suction. The fluence used was 12 J/cm² and the pulse duration was 60 ms. Both of the above subjects achieved excellent hair reduction and further benefit would likely be attained with additional treatments.

Table 4.1 Commercially available lasers and light sources for hair removal*

Laser/light source	Wavelength (nm)	System name	Pulse duration (ms)	Fluence (J/cm²)	Spot size (mm)	Other features
Long-pulsed ruby	694	RubyStar® and Ruby Star+® (Aesclepion, Germany)	4	Up to 24	8, 10, 12, 18	Contact cooling
Long-pulsed alexandrite	755	Apogee® (Cynosure, Westford, MA, USA)	0.5–300	2–50	5–15	Cold air or integrated cooling, can add 1064 nm Nd:YG module to form Apogee Elite®
		Arion® (Quantel Derma, Germany)	5–140	Up to 40	6–16	Cold air cooling
		ClearScan ALX® (Sciton, Palo Alto, CA, USA)	Up to 200	Up to 140	3, 6, and 30 × 30	Contact cooling

Continued

Table 4.1 Commercially available lasers and light sources for hair removal—cont'd

Laser/light source	Wavelength (nm)	System name	Pulse duration (ms)	Fluence (J/cm²)	Spot size (mm)	Other features
		Coolglide® (Cutera, Brisbane, CA, USA)	0.1–300	5–300	10	Contact cooling
		Elite® (Cynosure)	0.5–300	25–50	5–15	Cold air cooling, available with 1064 nm Nd:YAG, EliteMPX® model can simultaneously treat with 755 nm alexandrite and 1064 nm Nd:YAG
		EpiCare LP/LPX® (Light Age, Somerset, NJ, USA)	3–300	22–40	7–16	Dynamic cooling
		GentleLASE® (Syneron-Candela, Wayland, MA, USA) GentleMax® (Syneron-Candela)	3 0.25–300	Up to 100 Up to 600	6–18 1.5–18	Dynamic cooling, comes with 1064 Nd:YAG
		Ultrawave 755/II/III® (AMC Aesthetics and Advance Aesthetic Concepts, Plattsburgh, NY, USA)	Up to 100	Up to 125	Up to 16	Available with 532, 1064, and 1320 nm Nd:YAG
Diode	800–810	F1 Diode® (Opusmed, Canada)	15–40	Up to 40	5, 7	Chiller tip
	808, 980	Leda® (Quantel Derma)	6–60	Up to 60	50 × 12, 10 × 12	Contact cooling
	810, 940	MeDioStar XT® (Aesclepion)	5–500	Up to 90	6, 12	Integrated scanner with cold air cooling
	800	LightSheer Duet® (Lumenis, Israel)	5–400	10–100, 4.5–12	9 × 9, 22 × 35	Chilltip for smaller handpiece, vacuum skin flattening for larger handpiece
	810	Soprano XL® (Alma Lasers, Buffalo Grove, IL, USA)	10–1350	Up to 120	12 × 10	Contact cooling
Long-pulsed Nd:YAG	1064	Acclaim® (Cynosure)	0.4–300	35–600	1.5–15	Cold air or integrated cooling, can add 755 nm alexandrite module to form Apogee Elite® (Cynosure)
		ClearScan® YAG (Sciton)	0.3–200	Up to 400	3, 6, and 30 × 30	Contact cooling
		CoolGlide® CV/XEO/Excel/Vantage (Cutera)	0.1–300	Up to 300	3–10	Contact cooling
		Cynergy® (Cynosure)	0.3–300	Up to 600	1.5–15	Cold air
		SP and XP Dynamis®, XP Focus®, XP Max® (Fotona)	0.1–50	Up to 300	2–10	n/a
		GentleYAG® (Syneron-Candela, Wayland, MA)	0.25–300	Up to 600	1.5–18	Dynamic cooling
		Gemini® (Cutera)	1–-100	Up to 990	2, 10	Available with 532 nm KTP
		LightPod Neo® (Aerolase, Tarrytown, NY, USA)	0.65–1.5	Up to 312	2	

Table 4.1 Commercially available lasers and light sources for hair removal—cont'd

Laser/light source	Wavelength (nm)	System name	Pulse duration (ms)	Fluence (J/cm²)	Spot size (mm)	Other features
		Lyra® (Cutera)	20–100	5–900	1–5, 10	Built-in cooling system
		MultiFlex® (Ellipse, United Kingdom)	n/a	Up to 600	1.5–5	Contact cooling
		Mydon® (Quante Dermal)	0.5–90	10–450	1.5–10	Equipped with IPL device
		NaturaLase 1064/LP® (Focus Medical, Bethel, CT, USA)	0.5–100	Up to 400	3–15	Integrated air cooling
		Profile® (Sciton)	0.1–10000	Up to 75	n/a	Integrated air cooling
		SmartEpil® (Deka, Italy)	Up to 20	11	2.5, 4, 5, 6	Contact cooling, 2940 nm Er:YAG and 410–1400 nm flashlamp in same device
		Synchro_FT® (Deka)	2–30	Up to 50	2.5–13	Available with IPL handpiece
		Ultrawave II/III® (AMC Aesthetics, and Advance Aesthetic Concepts)	Up to 300	5–500	Up to 12	Pulsed cryogen cooling
		Varia® (CoolTouch, Roseville, CA, USA)	0.6	Up to 500	2–10	Dynamic cryogen cooling
Intense-pulsed light sources	520–1200	Axiom® (Viora, Jersey City, NJ, USA)	25–75 and 2.2–12.5	Up to 39	50 × 25, 35 × 15, 20 × 10	Built-in cooling system
	420–1400	BBL® (Sciton)	Up to 200	Up to 30	15 × 45	Built-in cooling system
	560–590	Cynergy® (Cynosure)	0.3–300	Up to 600	n/a	Built-in cooling system
	400–1200	Duet/SkinStation/SpaTouch II® (Radiancy. Orangeburg, NY, USA)	3–10	35	22 × 55	
	600–950	Ellipse I2PL/MultiFlex® (Ellipse)	2.5–88.5	4–26	10 × 48	
	650–950	Harmony XL® (Alma Lasers)	30–50	Up to 40	30 × 30	MultiFlex model with long-pulsed Nd:YAG
	530–1200	iPulse® (Dermavista, Birmingham, AL, USA)	10–110	Up to 20	8.9 sq cm	Available with 755 nm alexandrite and 1064 and 1320 nm Nd:YAG
	390–1200	Med Flash II® (General Project, Italy)	Up to 100	Up to 45	n/a	Air cooling
	525–1200	Icon/StarLux, R, Rs® (Palomar, Burlington, MA, USA)	5–500	Up to 70	28 × 12, 46 × 16	
	500–1200	MiniSilk_FT® (Deka)	3–8	Up to 160	48 × 13, 23 × 13	1064 nm Nd:YAG handpiece
	400–1200	Mistral® (Radiancy)	Up to 80	4–15	25 × 50, 13 × 50, 13 × 35, 12 × 12	Contact cooling

Continued

Table 4.1 Commercially available lasers and light sources for hair removal—cont'd

Laser/light source	Wavelength (nm)	System name	Pulse duration (ms)	Fluence (J/cm^2)	Spot size (mm)	Other features
	640–1400	NannoLight MP50® (Sybaritic, Minneapolis, MN, USA)	1–30	2.8–50	40 × 8	Nd:YAG handpiece, optional cooling
	640–1200	NaturaLight® (Solamed, Tampa, FL, USA)	Up to 500	Up to 50	10 × 40	
	750–1100	Solera Opus® (Cutera)	Auto	3–24	10 × 30	
	550–950	PhotoSilk Plus® (Deka)	Up to 30	10–340	21 × 10, 46 × 10, 46 × 18	
	770–1100	ProWave® (Cutera)	Auto	5–35	10 × 30	Nd:YAG handpiece
	500–1200	Quadra Q4® (DermaMed, Lenni, PA, USA)	48	10–20	33 × 15	
	695–1200	Quantum HR® (Lumenis)	15–100	25–45	34 × 8	
	560–950	SmoothCool® (Eclipse, Dallas, TX, USA)	1–60	10–45	8 × 34	Built-in cooling system
	530–1200	Trios® (Viora)	25	Up to 22	15 × 50	Automatic temperature control system
Fluorescent pulsed light	615–920	OmniLight/NovaLight® (American Medical Bio Care, Newport Beach, CA, USA)	2–500	Up to 90	7 × 15, 10 × 20, 30 × 30	Sapphire tip cooling
Optical energy combined with RF electrical energy	580–980	eMax/eLight® (Syneron)	Up to 100	Up to 50 optical; up to 50 J/cm^3 RF	12 × 15	Contact cooling
Diode combined with RF electrical energy	800	eLaser® (Syneron)	Up to 100	Up to 50 optical; up to 50 J/cm^3 RF	12 × 15	Contact cooling
	810	MeDioStar Effect® (Aesclepion)	Up to 500	Up to 90	10, 12, 14	Acoustic wave technology, integrated scanner with cold air cooling device, 940 nm simultaneously

*This table is intended only as a reference aid. The authors have made every attempt to provide an exhaustive list of available devices for laser hair removal but do not guarantee comprehensiveness.

laser treatment (Box 4.1). Patients with evidence of endocrine or menstrual dysfunction should be appropriately worked up. Similarly, patients with an explosive onset of hypertrichosis should be evaluated for paraneoplastic etiologies. Treatment of a pregnant woman for non-urgent conditions is discouraged by the authors, although there is no evidence suggesting a potential risk to pregnant women undergoing LHR. The past medical history should be reviewed to identify patients with photosensitive conditions, such as autoimmune connective tissue disorders, or disorders prone to the Koebner phenomenon. A history of recurrent cutaneous infections at or in the vicinity of the treatment area might warrant the use of prophylactic medications. Any past history of keloid or hypertrophic scar formation should be elicited as well. Previous hair removal methods, including past laser

Box 4.1
Pertinent medical history for laser/pulsed light hair removal

- Presence of conditions that may cause hypertrichosis:
- Hormonal
- Familial
- Drugs (i.e. corticosteroids, hormones, immunosuppressives, self or spousal use of minoxidil)
- Tumor
- History of local or recurrent skin infection
- History of herpes simplex, especially perioral
- History of herpes genitalis, important when treating the pubic or bikini area
- History of keloids/hypertrophic scarring
- History of koebnerizing skin disorders such as vitiligo and psoriasis
- Previous treatment modalities – method, frequency, and date of last treatment, as well as response
- Recent suntan or exposure to tanning or light cabinet
- Onset of hair regrowth (recent)
- Tattoos or nevi present
- Patient's expectations
- Patient's hobbies or habits which might interfere with treatment
- Present medications:
  - Photosensitizing medications
  - Isotretinoin intake within the past month

treatments, should be reviewed. Any methods of hair shaft epilation (e.g. waxing or tweezing) that entirely remove the target chromophore render LHR less effective for at least 2 weeks. Although there is little evidence for the time frame a patient must wait after complete epilation of the hair shaft and laser treatment, we recommend a minimum of 6 weeks. Shaving and depilatory creams can be used up to the day of laser treatment as they do not remove the entire hair shaft.

CASE STUDY 1

A 27-year-old Hispanic female with Fitzpatrick skin type IV presents to you for hair removal on the 'beard area'. She has been treated five times with a diode laser over the course of 2 years at a local spa and notes only a minimal reduction of hair. On review of systems, you discover that the patient has had a history of irregular menses and periodically flaring acne. She does not see a gynecologist.

While it appears that the patient is responding poorly to laser treatment, a thorough history reveals that the patient has clinical and historical evidence of hormonal dysfunction. This imbalance may be driving the conversion of vellus hair to terminal hair and can make it appear that laser hair removal treatments are ineffective, when in reality the patient is responding to treatment but is creating new hair follicles.

Pearl 1

It is imperative to counsel the patient not to partake in any epilation activities that remove the entire hair shaft. Shaving or using a chemical depilatory prior to treatment is acceptable but waxing or plucking will be counteractive to the laser treatments. A 2-week interval after such procedures is recommended for improved efficacy.

A medication history should be obtained. Gold intake is a contraindication for laser therapy with Q-switched lasers as there is a risk of the complication of chyrsiasis. The use of any photosensitizing medications or over-the-counter supplements should be held before treatment. Although there is a lack of convincing data, a washout period for patients on isotretinoin may be considered prior to laser treatment. Topical retinoids used in the treatment area should be discontinued 1 to 2 days prior to treatment. Finally, the patient's reaction to unprotected sun exposure (Fitzpatrick skin phototype) should be elicited as part of the history.

The physical exam should corroborate the patient's Fitzpatrick skin phototype. This will help determine which lasers and light sources are safe to use for that patient (see Table 4.1) because epidermal melanin in darkly pigmented patients competes with the melanin within hair follicles as a chromophore. Importantly, every patient should always be evaluated for the presence of a tan and, if present, laser treatment should be delayed or the treatment parameters appropriately adjusted until the tan has faded. Finally, the patient's hair color should be noted as the chromophore for LHR is melanin. Black and brown terminal hairs typically contain sufficient amount of melanin to serve as a chromophore for LHR. In contrast the lack of melanin, paucity of melanin or presence of eumelanin in the hair follicle, which clinically correlates with white, gray, or red/blonde hair respectively, is predictive of a poor response to laser hair removal (Fig. 4.3). For patients with little to no melanin in their hair follicles, attempts have been made to use exogenous chromophores that can be topically delivered to the hair follicles, thereby making the removal of white, gray, red, and blonde hair hypothetically possible. This concept was first demonstrated with a topical carbon solution dissolved in mineral oil. However, we have noticed very little long-term hair reduction efficacy of topical chromophores in our experience. The coarseness and density of hair are also important to note as these factors will influence parameter settings (see below).

Pearl 2

Treatment on tanned patients should be delayed until the tan fades. Risk of pigmentary alteration is significantly higher in these patients.

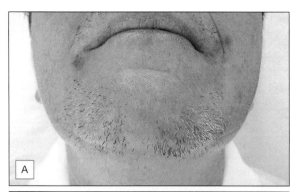

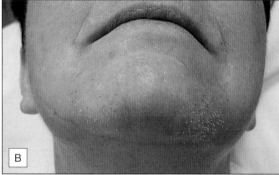

Figure 4.3 Effective laser hair removal can be obtained for dark, pigmented hairs, but not for white hairs: (**A**) before, and (**B**) after treatment.

> **Pearl 3**
>
> Patients with white, gray, or blonde hair are currently not appropriate candidates for laser hair removal. Other methods of epilation should be encouraged.

Informed consent

Informed consent requires a review of the potential risks of LHR, which include, but are not limited to, temporary and permanent hypo/hyperpigmentation, blister formation, scar formation, ulceration, hive-like response, bruising, infection, acne flare, and folliculitis. For those patients with Fitzpatrick skin type IV or greater or of Mediterranean, Middle Eastern, Asian or South Asian descent, the low risk of paradoxical hypertrichosis (conversion of vellus hairs to thicker, more obvious terminal hairs), especially when treating the lateral face and jaw, should be reviewed. Patients should be counseled that permanent and complete hair removal is not likely but that, with multiple treatments, significant long-term reduction can be achieved. Hirsute women with hormonal abnormalities such as polycystic ovarian syndrome may require continued maintenance therapy and should be advised of this possibility. Procedural pain is expected with LHR but can be minimized with topical anesthetics. Erythema and edema are also expected with treatment and may last up to 1 week. Patients should be aware of the need for strict sun avoidance for a minimum of 6 weeks before and after each treatment.

> **CASE STUDY 2**
>
> A 32-year old Egyptian female presents for laser hair removal of the lateral preauricular face. On physical exam, she is a Fitzpatrick skin type V with fine, dark vellus hairs in the area of interest.
>
> This patient is a challenge for a variety of reasons (dark skin type, caliber of hair to be treated). Importantly, it is critical for the laser surgeon to also review the rare risk of paradoxical hypertrichosis (see above). Paradoxical hypertrichosis is a poorly understood phenomenon in which laser stimulates hair growth or a change in hair type from vellus to terminal hairs. This produces an obvious worsening in the appearance of the affected hairs in a cosmetically sensitive area, i.e. the face. Although challenging, these increased hairs can be treated with further hair removal but they may be more resistant to therapy.

Preoperative preparation and laser safety

The need for topical anesthesia is variable among patients and anatomic sites. Various topical anesthetics including lidocaine, lidocaine/prilocaine, and other amide/ester anesthetic combinations can be used to diminish the procedural discomfort, and should be applied 30 minutes to 1 hour before treatment under occlusion. Care should be taken when using lidocaine or prilocaine to apply these medications to a limited area to diminish the risk of lidocaine toxicity or methemoglobulinemia, respectively. Deaths have resulted from lidocaine toxicity resulting from occlusion of the back as well as lower extremities with topical lidocaine. Likewise, systemic toxicity can occur with the use of any topical anesthetic in large amounts.

> **Pearl 4**
>
> Occlusion increases the absorption of topical medications by at least an order of magnitude. Lidocaine is a cardiotoxic medication and prilocaine can convert hemoglobin into methemoglobulin. Large areas such as the back or legs should have topical anesthesia applied with caution.

Patients should be placed in a room with a treatment chair that makes the desired treatment area easily accessible. The room should be adequately cooled to keep the laser device from overheating and be free of any hanging mirrors or uncovered windows. A fire extinguisher should be readily available. If possible, supplemental oxygen should be turned off when performing laser treatments. Having a vacuum device on hand during treatment can minimize the plume and unpleasant odor created by each laser pulse. Because the retina contains melanin that can be damaged by wavelengths in the red and near-infrared range, proper eye protection is absolutely critical for both the patient and laser surgeon. Goggles are not interchangeable between lasers or IPL devices of different wavelengths. Furthermore, because of the risk of retinal damage from the deeply penetrating wavelengths used for LHR, one should never treat a patient for LHR within the bony orbit.

CASE STUDY 3

A 35-year old female with Fitzpatrick skin type II and jet-black hair presents to you for laser hair removal. During the consultation, she states her primary concern is that she would like to have her eyebrows shaped permanently. She is inconvenienced by her current regimen of waxing every several weeks.

The patient is an ideal candidate for LHR with her fair skin and dark hair. Almost any hair removal laser would be appropriate for use. The issue of concern in this case is the location of treatment. Caution must be taken when treating near the eye, as there is a risk of damage to retinal pigment.

Device variables

Wavelength

The chromophore for laser hair removal is melanin. Within the hair follicle, melanin is principally located within the hair shaft, although the outer root sheath and matrix area also contain melanin. Melanin is capable of functioning as a chromophore for wavelengths in the red and near-IR portion of the electromagnetic spectrum, and can be targeted by ruby, alexandrite, diode and Nd:YAG lasers, as well as IPL devices.

The long-pulsed ruby laser (694 nm) was the first device used to selectively target hair follicles, resulting in long-term hair loss. The long-pulsed ruby laser can be safely used in Fitzpatrick skin phototypes I–III. Table 4.1 lists the long-pulsed ruby lasers that are commercially available.

The long-pulsed alexandrite (755 nm) laser has been shown to be effective for long-term hair removal in multiple studies. The long-pulsed alexandrite laser can be safely used in Fitzpatrick skin phototypes I–IV, although some experts limit the use of the long-pulsed alexandrite laser to Fitzpatrick skin phototypes I–III. A few studies have demonstrated the safety of the long-pulsed alexandrite laser in a large cohort of patients with Fitzpatrick skin phototypes IV–VI. Combination treatment of alexandrite and Nd:YAG lasers provides no added benefit over the alexandrite laser alone. The commercially available long-pulsed alexandrite devices are summarized in Table 4.1.

The long-pulsed diode (800–810 nm) laser (LPDL) has also been extensively used for LHR. The diode laser can be safely used in patients with Fitzpatrick skin phototypes I–V and has good long-term efficacy for LHR.

The long-pulsed Nd:YAG laser has been thought to offer the best combination of safety and efficacy for

Fitzpatrick skin phototype VI patients. Long-term hair reduction with 18-month follow-up showed 73.6% clearance following four treatments at 2-month intervals.

IPL is composed of polychromatic, non-coherent light ranging from 400 to 1200 nm. Various filters can be used to target particular chromophores, including melanin. Long-term (>1 year) hair removal has not been convincingly demonstrated to date. Various reports have demonstrated short-term efficacy. One study of patients treated with a single IPL session reported 75% hair removal 1 year after treatment. Two studies providing a head-to-head comparison of IPL versus either the long-pulsed alexandrite laser or Nd:YAG laser both found the IPL to be inferior to laser devices for hair removal. In contrast, a study of hirsute women, some with a diagnosis of polycystic ovarian syndrome, who underwent a split-face treatment with six IPL or LDPL show statistically equivalent reductions in hair counts at 1 (77% versus 68%, respectively), 3 (53% versus 60%, respectively) and 6 months (40% versus 34%, respectively) after the final treatment.

Pearl 5

One should always evaluate the patient's Fitzpatrick skin type when evaluating a patient for LHR. Darker skin types require longer wavelengths, which pose a lower risk of side effects from the absorption of energy by epidermal melanin.

Fluence

Fluence is defined as the amount of energy delivered per unit area and is expressed as J/cm^2. Higher fluences have been correlated with greater permanent hair removal, but are also more likely to cause untoward side effects. Recommended treatment fluences are often provided with each individual laser device for non-experienced operators. However, a more appropriate method of determining the optimal treatment fluence for a given patient is to evaluate for the desired clinical end point of perifollicular erythema and edema seen within a few minutes of treatment (Fig. 4.4). The highest possible tolerated fluence that yields this end point without any adverse effects is the best fluence for treatment. Fluences that cause epidermal disruption are too high and should be reduced.

Pearl 6

When treating a patient for LHR for the first time, it may be prudent to try several test spots at varying fluences to determine the optimal settings. The highest tolerable fluence without epidermal damage will yield the greatest amount of hair clearance per treatment.

Pulse duration

Pulse duration is defined as the duration in seconds of laser exposure. The theory of selective photothermolysis

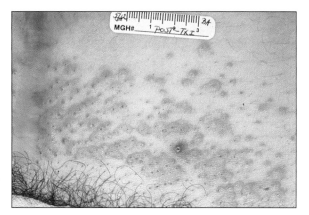

Figure 4.4 Formation of perifollicular eythema and edema immediately after laser treatment.

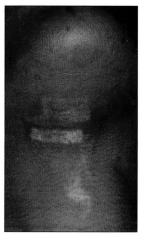

Figure 4.5 Inadequate contact cooling resulting in postinflammatory hypopigmentation in a patient with type V skin. *Photograph courtesy of Nathan Uebelhoer.*

enables the laser surgeon to select an optimal pulse duration based on the thermal relaxation time (TRT). Terminal hairs are about 300 μm in diameter, and thus the calculated TRT of a terminal hair follicle is about 100 ms. However, unlike many other laser applications, the hair follicle is distinct in that there is a spatial separation of the chromophore (melanin) within the hair shaft and the biological 'target' stem cells in the bulge and bulb areas of the follicle. The expanded theory of selective photothermolysis takes this spatial separation into account and proposes a thermal damage time (TDT), which is longer than the TRT. Shorter pulse widths are also capable of removing hair, and it is unclear which is more effective in producing permanent hair removal. Longer pulse widths are likely more selective for melanin within the hair follicle and can minimize epidermal damage as the pulse widths are greater than the TRT of the melanosomes in epidermal keratinocytes and melanocytes.

Pearl 7

When treating darker Fitzpatrick skin types, a longer pulse duration is preferred as the pulse duration exceeds the thermal relaxation time of the epidermal melanin, and minimizes the risk of epidermal damage.

Spot size

The spot size is the diameter in millimeters of the laser beam. As photons within a laser beam penetrate the dermis they are scattered by collagen fibers, and those that are scattered outside the area of the laser beam are essentially wasted. Photons are more likely to be scattered outside of the beam area for smaller spot sizes, whereas in a larger spot size the photons are likely to remain within the beam area following scatter. A double-blind, randomized controlled trial of a long-pulsed alexandrite laser for LHR of the axillary region comparing 18 and 12 mm spot sizes at otherwise identical treatment parameters showed a 10% greater reduction in hair counts with the larger spot

size. Recently, a prospective study using a LDPL with a large 22 × 35 mm handpiece at low fluences and no skin cooling was shown to have similar long-term hair removal efficacy to published studies of LPDLs with smaller spot sizes using higher fluences and skin cooling. Thus, larger spot sizes are preferable to smaller spot sizes.

Pearl 8

Using the largest possible spot size allows for optimal penetration and minimizes the number of pulses it takes to cover a treatment area, thereby translating to faster treatment courses.

Skin cooling

The presence of epidermal melanin, particularly in darker skin types, presents a competing chromophore to hair follicle melanin, which can be damaged during LHR (Fig. 4.5). Cooling of the skin surface is used to minimize epidermal damage as well as pain, while permitting treatment with higher fluences. All of the skin-cooling methods function by acting as a heat sink and removing heat from the skin surface. The least effective type of cooling is the use of an aqueous cold gel, which passively extracts heats from the skin and then is not capable of further skin cooling. Alternatively, cooling with forced chilled air can provide cooling to the skin before, during, and after a laser pulse. Currently, most of the available LHR devices have a built-in skin cooling system, which consists of either contact cooling or dynamic cooling with a cryogen spray. Contact cooling, usually with a sapphire tip, provides skin cooling just before and during a laser pulse. It is most useful for treatments with longer pulse durations (>10 ms). Dynamic cooling with cryogen liquid spray precools the skin with a millisecond spray of cryogen just before the laser pulse. A second spray can be delivered just after the laser pulse for post-cooling, but parallel cooling during the laser pulse is not possible as the cryogen spray interferes with the laser beam. Dynamic cooling is best suited for use with pulse durations shorter than 5 ms.

Pearl 9

Skin cooling is beneficial for minimizing epidermal damage and treatment-associated pain. However, cooling can be overdone and result in pigmentary alterations, particularly with cryogen liquid spray.

Post-procedure care

It is expected for the patient to have perifollicular erythema and edema in the treatment area following LHR. This generally persists for 2 days but can last for up to 1 week. Ice and application of a topical corticosteroid can be used to shorten the duration of these undesired clinical findings. Patients will often find that a single treatment of LHR with shorter pulse durations results in nearly total epilation of the hair follicles in the treatment area. It is important to counsel the patient that a majority of these hairs will likely regrow, and this isn't considered a treatment failure. Generally, only about 15% of hairs are permanently removed with each laser treatment. On the other hand, LHR treatments with longer pulse durations may leave behind many hairs that appear to 'grow' following treatment. It is important to reassure the patient that these 'growing' hairs are dislodged from the hair follicle and require 1–2 weeks to be completely shed. Nearly any method of epilation can be used to hasten their removal.

The importance of strict sun precaution following LHR treatments cannot be overemphasized. This can be achieved by the use of topical sunscreens, ultraviolet light impermeable garments, and, most importantly, sun avoidance.

Pearl 10

Beyond SPF30, higher SPF values do not necessarily correlate with increased protection from the sun. The SPF value of a product only reflects its protection from UVB rays. It is far more important that the product contain broad-spectrum protection, including UVA rays.

Long-term efficacy

Evidence of permanent hair removal was evident as early as the seminal hair removal trial from the Wellman Center involving a single treatment with the normal mode ruby laser. Seven of the 13 original subjects were evaluated at 2-year follow-up. Of the 7 subjects, 4 had evidence of persistent permanent hair reduction at 2-year follow-up, whereas 3 subjects experienced complete regrowth. Follow-up of 18 out of the 50 original study subjects treated with a LPDL showed a 25–33% and 36–46% hair reduction at a mean follow-up of 20 months after one

or two treatments (9 mm spot size, pulse duration of 5–20 ms, fluences of 15–40 J/cm^2, single or triple pulsed) respectively. A head-to-head trial comparing a LPDL to a long-pulsed alexandrite laser found a 49–94% hair reduction at 1-year follow-up after four treatments (9 mm spot size, pulse duration of 20 ms, fluences of 12–40 J/cm^2) with the LPDL in 15 subjects. Similar results were achieved with the alexandrite laser used in this study. Fifteen of 20 subjects with Fitzpatrick skin phototypes III–IV treated with a long-pulsed alexandrite laser (12 and 18 mm spot size, 3 ms pulse duration and fluences of 20 or 40 J/cm^2) or a long-pulsed Nd:YAG laser (12 mm spot size, 3 ms pulse duration and fluence of 40 J/cm^2) for four sessions at 8-week intervals showed 76–84% and 74% hair reduction 18 months after the last treatment respectively. Another head-to-head trial of a high fluence LPDL (9 mm spot size, pulse duration of 30 ms, fluences of 20–50 J/cm^2) versus a low fluence LPDL (12 × 10 mm spot size, pulse duration of 20 ms, fluences of 5–10 J/cm^2) in 22 subjects showed similar, 94% and 90% hair reduction at 18 month follow-up following five treatments spaced 6–8 weeks apart, respectively. Finally, the authors recently reported statistically significant hair clearance, 54% and 42%, at 6- and 15-month follow-up visits following three monthly treatments using a LPDL with a large handpiece in the largest prospective trial to date. Remaining hairs were found to also grow back less thick and lighter.

Complications

The most common complications of LHR are epidermal damage (Fig. 4.6) and pigmentary alterations, including hyper- and hypopigmentation (Fig. 4.7). This may result from selecting a non-optimal wavelength, pulse duration or fluence, using inadequate epidermal cooling or treating a tanned patient (Fig. 4.8). Pigmentary alterations may also occur even when optimal treatment parameters are used. These changes are often transient and improve with time, although permanent hypopigmentation can occur

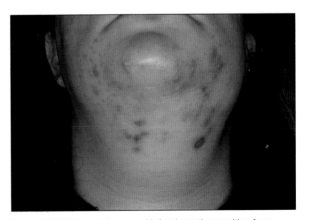

Figure 4.6 Epidermal damage with focal crusting resulting from excessive laser fluence.

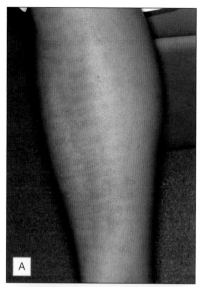

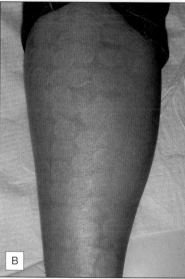

Figure 4.7 Example of laser hair removal induced hyperpigmentation (**A**) and permanent hypopigmentation (**B**).

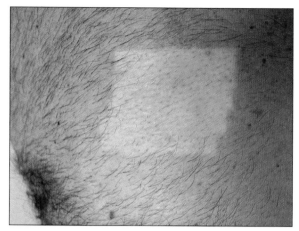

Figure 4.8 Treatment of recently tanned skin resulted in development of hypopigmentation.

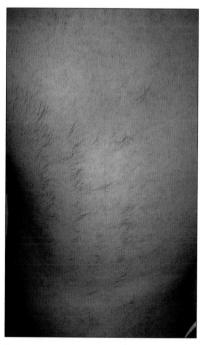

Figure 4.9 Zones of untreated skin resulting from lack of appropriate overlapping.

(Fig. 4.7B). Zones of untreated hairs can result from a lack of overlapping between laser pulses (Fig. 4.9). Scarring is an exceedingly rare complication but can occur when excessive fluences and/or pulse stacking are used.

Treatment of the lateral cheeks and chin area, or less commonly other areas, may result in the induction of terminal hairs, a phenomenon known as paradoxical hypertrichosis (Fig. 4.10). This has been reported to occur more commonly in females of Mediterranean, Middle Eastern, Asian and South Asian descent. The exact mechanism remains uncharacterized but it is thought that sub-therapeutic laser fluences may lead to the stimulation of hair growth.

Caution should be exercised to avoid treatment of tattoos and nevi, particularly atypical nevi.

Future directions

Advances in pain control

A novel technique to reduce LHR-associated pain is pneumatic skin flattening (PSF). PSF works by coupling a vacuum chamber to generate negative pressure and to flatten the skin against the hand piece treatment window. Based on the gate theory of pain transmission, it stimulates pressure receptors in the skin immediately prior to

Notably, none of the subjects in the study reported experiencing severe or intolerable pain.

Home-use laser and light source devices for hair removal

In recent years, a number of devices have been developed that seek to provide patients with the ability to achieve energy-based hair removal at home. These devices are based on intense pulsed light (IPL), laser and thermal technologies that target the hair follicle for destruction. Devices that have 510(k) clearance by the Federal Drug Administration (FDA) in the United States include: (1) thermal-based devices (no!no!hair® [Radiancy, Orangeburg, NY]); (2) IPL-based devices including Silkn SensEpil® (Skinnovations, Israel) and Viss IPL® (Viss Beauty, Korea); (3) laser-based devices (Tria Laser 3.0® [Tria Beauty, Pleasanton, CA]); and (4) combined IPL/thermal-based devices including the SpaTouch Elite® and Kona® (Radiancy). Similar technologies are also being utilized by a variety of other home use devices that do not currently have FDA 510(k) clearance.

The evidence behind such devices is scant and limited to small non-controlled studies. In addition, the risk for devastating eye injuries with improper use of laser- and IPL-based devices and lack of medical training raises a dilemma of how much autonomy a patient should have with potentially harmful devices. None the less, the appeal of having a personal device to remove unwanted hair in the privacy of one's home without the expense and inconvenience of multiple dermatologist or spa visits will likely drive the development of additional home use devices.

Alternative technologies for hair removal

Photodynamic therapy (PDT) with aminolevulinic acid (ALA) has been shown in a small pilot study to result in up to 40% hair reduction with a single treatment, although wax epilation was performed prior to treatment in this study.

Electro-optical synergy (ELOS) technology combines electrical (conducted radiofrequency) and optical (laser/light) energies. A handful of devices based on this technology have been produced (see Table 4.1). The theory behind ELOS is based on the optical component (laser or IPL) heating the hair shaft, which then is thought to concentrate the bipolar radiofrequency (RF) energy to the surrounding hair follicle. Based on this combination, lower fluences are needed for the optical component, thereby suggesting it might be well tolerated in all Fitzpatrick skin phototypes, and potentially effective in the removal of white and poorly pigmented hair. A study of 40 patients (Fitzpatrick skin phenotypes II–V) with varied facial and non-facial hair colors were treated with combined IPL/RF ELOS technology. An average clearance of 75% was observed at 18 months following four treatments. No significant adverse sequelae were noted and there were no treatment differences between patients of varying skin types or hair color. Pre-treatment with aminolevulinic acid

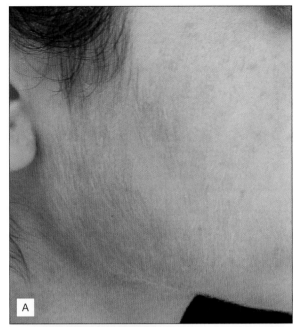

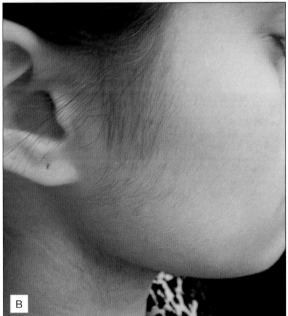

Figure 4.10 Paradoxical hypertrichosis. Conversion of fine, vellus-like hairs (**A**) to terminal dark hairs (**B**) after a single laser hair removal treatment.

firing of the laser pulse, thereby blocking activation of pain fibers. PSF is just beginning to be incorporated into commercially available lasers (see Table 4.1). A recent study of LHR using a LPDL with a large spot size and vacuum-assisted suction showed that the majority of subjects reported feeling no pain at all or up to moderate pain without the use of skin cooling or topical anesthetics.

(ALA) prior to use of a combined IPL and radiofrequency device has been shown to further augment the removal of terminal white hairs.

In conclusion, hair removal has made a dramatic shift from an art to science based on the theory of selective photothermolysis. Since the first reports of selective hair removal in 1996 by Anderson and colleagues, there has been a tremendous explosion in the number of devices used for LHR, making LHR the most commonly requested cosmetic procedure in the world. This chapter provides the reader with the fundamentals of hair follicle anatomy and physiology, points for patient selection and preoperative preparation, principles of laser safety, an introduction to the various laser/light devices and a discussion of laser–tissue interactions that are vital to optimizing treatment efficacy while minimizing complications and side effects.

Further reading

Alster TS, Bryan H, Williams CM 2001 Long-pulsed Nd:YAG laser-assisted hair removal in pigmented skin: a clinical and histological evaluation. Archives of Dermatology 137(7): 885-889

Altshuler GB, Anderson RR, Manstein D, et al 2001 Extended theory of selective photothermolysis. Lasers in Surgery and Medicine 29(5):416-432

Anderson RR, Parrish JA 1983 Selective photothermolysis: precise microsurgery by selective absorption of pulsed radiation. Science 220(4596):524-527

Bernstein EF 2005 Hair growth induced by diode laser treatment. Dermatologic Surgery 31(5):584-586

Braun M 2011 Comparison of high-fluence, single-pass diode laser to low-fluence, multiple-pass diode laser for laser hair reduction with 18 months of follow up. Journal of Drugs in Dermatology 10(1):62-65

Campos VB, Dierickx CC, Farinelli WA, et al 2000 Hair removal with an 800-nm pulsed diode laser. Journal of the American Academy of Dermatology 43(3):442-447

Davoudi SM, Behnia F, Gorouhi F, et al 2008 Comparison of long-pulsed alexandrite and Nd:YAG lasers, individually and in combination, for leg hair reduction: an assessor-blinded, randomized trial with 18 months of follow-up. Archives of Dermatology 144(10):1323-1327

Dierickx CC, Grossman MC, Farinelli WA, et al 1998 Permanent hair removal by normal-mode ruby laser. Archives of Dermatology 134(7):837-842

Eremia S, Li C, Newman N 2001 Laser hair removal with alexandrite versus diode laser using four treatment sessions: 1-year results. Dermatologic Surgery 27(11):925-929; discussion 929-930

Garcia C, Alamoudi H, Nakib M, et al 2000 Alexandrite laser hair removal is safe for Fitzpatrick skin types IV–VI. Dermatologic Surgery 26(2):130-134

Gold MH, Bell MW, Foster TD, et al 1999 One-year follow-up using an intense pulsed light source for long-term hair removal. Journal of Cutaneous Laser Therapy 1(3):167-171

Goldberg DJ, Littler CM, Wheeland RG 1997 Topical suspension-assisted Q-switched Nd:YAG laser hair removal. Dermatologic Surgery 23(9):741-745

Grossman MC, Dierickx C, Farinelli W, et al 1996 Damage to hair follicles by normal-mode ruby laser pulses. Journal of the American Academy of Dermatology 35(6):889-894

Haak CS, Nymann P, Pedersen AT, et al 2010 Hair removal in hirsute women with normal testosterone levels: a randomized controlled trial of long-pulsed diode laser vs. intense pulsed light. British Journal of Dermatology 163(5):1007-1013

Hussain M, Polnikorn N, Goldberg DJ 2003 Laser-assisted hair removal in Asian skin: efficacy, complications, and the effect of single versus multiple treatments. Dermatologic Surgery 29(3):249-254

Ibrahimi OA, Avram MM, Hanke CW, et al 2011 Laser hair removal. Dermatologic Therapy 24(1):94-107

Ibrahimi OA, Kilmer SL 2012 Long-term clinical evaluation of a 800 nm long-pulsed diode laser with a large spot size and vacuum-assisted suction for hair removal. Dermatologic Surgery 38(6):912-917

Khoury JG, Saluja R, Goldman MP 2008 Comparative evaluation of long-pulse alexandrite and long-pulse Nd:YAG laser systems used individually and in combination for axillary hair removal. Dermatologic Surgery 34(5):665-670; discussion 670-661

Lask G, Friedman D, Elman M, et al 2006 Pneumatic skin flattening (PSF): a novel technology for marked pain reduction in hair removal with high energy density lasers and IPLs. Journal of Cosmetic and Laser Therapy 8(2):76-81

Lou WW, Quintana AT, Geronemus RG, et al 2000 Prospective study of hair reduction by diode laser (800 nm) with long-term follow-up. Dermatologic Surgery 26(5):428-432

Nouri K, Chen H, Saghari S, et al 2004 Comparing 18- versus 12-mm spot size in hair removal using a gentlease 755-nm alexandrite laser. Dermatologic Surgery 30(4 Pt 1):494-497

Rao J, Goldman MP 2005 Prospective, comparative evaluation of three laser systems used individually and in combination for axillary hair removal. Dermatologic Surgery 31(12):1671-1676; discussion 1677

Richards RN, Meharg GE 1885 Electrolysis: observations from 13 years and 140,000 hours of experience. Journal of the American Academy of Dermatology 33(4):662-666

Rohrer TE, Chatrath V, Yamauchi P, et al 2003 Can patients treat themselves with a small novel light based hair removal system? Lasers in Surgery and Medicine 33(1):25-29

Zenzie HH, Altshuler GB, Smirnov MZ, et al 2000 Evaluation of cooling methods for laser dermatology. Lasers in Surgery and Medicine 26(2):130-144

Non-ablative laser and light skin rejuvenation

Travis W. Blalock, E. Victor Ross

5

Summary and Key Features

- Non-ablative skin resurfacing is a safe and effective means of improving many aspects of photoaged skin
- While non-ablative skin resurfacing provides modest results, it also provides minimal downtime
- Non-ablative resurfacing alters cellular and non-cellular components of the skin without causing an open wound
- Patient selection requires careful consideration of medical factors as well as patient expectations
- Non-ablative modalities rarely require more than local anesthesia
- When performed with thoughtful consideration, complications are rare
- Photodynamic therapy has been utilized to maximize laser–tissue interaction and subsequent improvement in photoaging
- Treatment of types IV–VI skin requires adjustment of laser parameters to minimize pigment alteration
- Patients can generally return to their normal activities in 1–2 days following treatment with non-ablative modalities
- For patients with limited available downtime, multiple treatments 2–3 months apart may provide an improved result

Introduction

With the advancement of laser and non-laser light sources, the focus of skin rejuvenation is optimizing efficacy while minimizing recovery times. The gold standard for rejuvenation, at least for fine wrinkles, has been ablative modalities. Although ablative tools can achieve predictable cosmetic enhancement, the risks of scarring, infection, dyspigmentation, and prolonged recovery time make these modalities less attractive. Patients increasingly try to balance efficacy of skin rejuvenation within the context of downtime. Non-ablative skin rejuvenation normally mitigates the need for advanced anesthesia and can often be performed with only topical anesthesia. Thus, non-ablative modalities have enjoyed a greater role in skin rejuvenation.

A clear definition of non-ablative skin rejuvenation is important as the term is sometimes used haphazardly. In its most pure form, non-ablative rejuvenation improves skin quality without physical removal or vaporization of the skin. Ablative modalities, via vaporization, remove a portion, or all, of the epidermis and sometimes may remove parts of the dermis. This chapter focuses exclusively on non-fractional methods of non-ablative skin rejuvenation.

The dermis (and/or deeper epidermis) can be selectively damaged by two basic approaches:

1. Targeting discrete chromophores in the dermis and/or at the dermal epidermal junction, or
2. Using mid-infrared lasers in the range of 1.3–1.55 µm wavelengths, where water absorption is weak enough that relatively deep beam penetration is allowed (there is only 50% beam attenuation at depths of 300–1500 µm).

Treatment of photodamage can be divided into various categories, and treatment protocols are based on a logical approach founded on the laser–tissue interactions delineated above. The goal should be to maximize skin rejuvenation, from reducing telangiectasias and lentigines to enhancing dermal remodeling.

The laser and non-laser systems used for non-ablative rejuvenation are a heterogeneous group of devices that emit wavelengths in the visible (400–760 nm), near-infrared (760–1400 nm), or mid-infrared (1.4–3 µm) ranges, radiofrequency (RF) devices, intense pulsed light (IPL) devices, as well as light-emitting diode (LED) devices (Box 5.1). Each of these modalities can induce dermal remodeling, as well as target other components, without epidermal ablation. Most investigators believe that photothermal heating of the dermis: (1) increases collagen production by fibroblasts and (2) induces dermal matrix remodeling by altering glycosaminoglycans as well as other components of the dermal matrix. Others believe that the laser/light interaction with molecular cellular components alters the cellular function of enzymes as well as cellular structural components. Altering the different components of cells, from enzymes to cellular wall

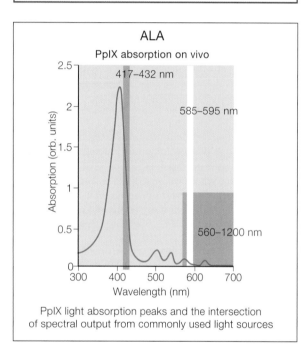

ALA

PpIX absorption on vivo

PpIX light absorption peaks and the intersection of spectral output from commonly used light sources

Figure 5.1 Protoporphyrin IX absorption: due to the multiple absorption peaks of protoporphyrin IX, multiple lasers and light sources can be used to augment the effects following application of porphyrin precursors to the skin.

constituents to nucleic acids, may then alter the environment and productivity of a given cell.

Photodynamic therapy (PDT) with aminolevulinic acid (ALA) has been show to augment the effects of laser or other light sources. Multiple laser and light sources have been used for photoactivation of protoporphyrin IX, leading to improved skin rejuvenation (Fig. 5.1).

Non-ablative skin rejuvenation is commonly used to reverse photoaging in the dermis. This damage is directly correlated with the patient's age and extent of ultraviolet exposure. Ultraviolet B (UVB) light alters nucleic acids as it interacts with epidermal keratinocytes, inducing cellular atypia. Over time, longer-wavelength ultraviolet A (UVA) light causes increases in oxygen radical formation, inducing alterations in the normal homeostasis of vessel formation, apoptosis, pigment generation by melanocytes, immune cell dysregulation, cytokine dysregulation, alteration of dermal matrix composition, and disruption in the transcription, translation, and replication of the cellular genetic code. Histological changes that accompany the clinical findings of photoaging include an atrophic epidermis, loss of the rete pattern, elastic fiber clumping in the papillary dermis, haphazard and reduced collagen production, and increased vasculature. These UV-induced changes correlate with the clinical appearance of photoaged skin, including skin laxity, atrophy and fragility, increased rhytid formation, telangiectasia, and alteration in the overall color, texture, and consistency of the skin. Thus the goal of rejuvenation is to replace damaged epidermal or dermal constituents with more robust, newly created ones. Physicians attempt to alter the quality of the keratinocytes and the pigment production of melanocytes, two key components of epidermal photodamage. Dermal photodamage rejuvenation typically has concentrated on improving the quality and inhibiting the degeneration of fibroblasts. Studies have shown an increase in antioxidant capacity and collagen synthesis after millisecond and nanosecond 532 nm and 1064 nm laser irradiation in fibroblast cell cultures.

Richard Glogau, MD developed a classification scale to chart the progression of clinical photoaging (Table 5.1). One can follow a patient from an early age, with relatively strong homogeneity of skin coloration and minimal wrinkles, to a more aged patient, with wrinkles at rest and a more heterogeneous skin coloration.

As one would expect, treating a Glogau grade I patient with current non-ablative modalities will achieve a higher percentage of photoaging correction versus more severely photodamaged patients. While ablative skin rejuvenation may achieve superior restoration of normal skin structures, especially for the Glogau grade III or IV patient (see Table 5.1), the downtime and potential risks are prohibitive for many patients. Nevertheless, as non-ablative technologies evolve, restoration of young, healthy skin with diminished risks and negligible recovery times is increasingly possible. The remainder of the chapter will focus on patient selection for non-ablative skin rejuvenation and discussion of the different devices.

Patient selection

Patient selection for non-ablative skin rejuvenation begins with an assessment of the degree and type of photoaging (see Table 5.1). The ideal patient is Glogau grade II or III with mild to moderate photodamage. Non-ablative therapies initiate new collagen formation (collagen I and collagen III) and might be appropriate in a Glogau grade I patient to prevent photodamage progression. Alternatively, a patient and/or a physician expecting dramatic

Table 5.1 Glogau photoaging classification

Grade	Classification	Typical age	Description	Skin characteristics
I	Mild	20s or 30s	No wrinkles	Early photoaging: mild pigmentary change, no keratoses, minimal wrinkles, minimal or no makeup
II	Moderate	30s or 40s	Wrinkles in motion	Early to moderate photoaging: early solar lentigines, keratoses palpable but not visible, parallel smile lines begin to appear, wears some foundation
III	Advanced	50s	Wrinkles at rest	Advanced photoaging: obvious discolorations, visible telangiectasias, visible keratoses, wears heavier foundation always
IV	Severe	60s and older	Only wrinkles	Severe photoaging: yellow-gray skin color, prior skin malignancies, wrinkles throughout – no normal skin, makeup 'cakes and cracks'

change following a non-ablative rejuvenation procedure in a Glogau grade IV patient may be disappointed.

Sadick divides patients in a different manner, where cosmetic deficiencies are based on the histological location of solar damage. His selection process takes into account epidermal (type I) damage (Fig. 5.2) and dermal/subcutaneous (type II) damage (Fig. 5.3), and subsequently treatment is tailored to laser selectivity of the damage.

Another important factor in patient selection is the patient's Fitzpatrick skin type. Fitzpatrick IV, V, and VI skin types may not be optimal candidates for particular non-ablative rejuvenation modalities that selectively heat melanin. The most common adverse result for non-ablative rejuvenation in darker skin patients is hyperpigmentation, a condition that usually resolves after 4–8 weeks (but can persist longer in some circumstances) with appropriate application of suppressors of melanin synthesis. Mid-infrared lasers, which minimize direct melanin targeting, can be used in patients with darker skin types. However, higher fluences in these patients may result in thermal damage and bulk heating, which can also result in dyspigmentation. Non-cryogen cooling devices can minimize bulk heating, whereas cooling devices that employ cryogen spray may induce pigmentary alterations similar to liquid nitrogen. See Chapter 10 for a detailed discussion of laser and non-laser light sources for the treatment of darker skin types.

Beyond skin type and amount of photodamage, there are some patients who might be excluded from non-ablative lasers and light sources based on medical criteria (Box 5.2). Oral retinoid use, recent rejuvenation procedures, infection, and active dermatitides are reasons to consider deferring a non-ablative rejuvenation procedure. Most likely oral retinoids will not affect the outcome, but no controlled study has investigated their effect on non-ablative skin resurfacing. Many texts advocate waiting a period of 6–12 months, most likely representing an extrapolation from ablative resurfacing wait times. Some cutaneous laser experts have used non-ablative devices 1 month following retinoid use without adverse outcomes.

Physicians must also consider the wavelength of the device. For example, devices that utilize visible light (i.e. LED devices, etc.) may exacerbate a phototoxicity/photosensitivity or a systemic condition that is photosensitive, like cutaneous lupus (although in a recent study only 7% of SLE patients reacted to visible light) (Fig. 5.4). On the other hand, some lasers may confer a protective quality. There is increasing evidence that IPL can activate fibroblasts as well as confer protection from future UV-induced skin damage.

Fillers and neurotoxins most likely are not affected by non-ablative modalities and can be administered in the same session. However, the non-ablative resurfacing should be performed last. This order will minimize the risk of neurotoxin diffusion, which should cease by 1 hour after the injection, and will reduce the possibility of edema obscuring endpoints in optimal filler placement.

Visible light and near-infrared/vascular lasers (Table 5.2)

Visible light lasers and near-infrared lasers are commonly used to treat vascular and pigmented lesions. Treatment of vascular lesions with visible light lasers can achieve histological correction of dyspigmentation, overall skin texture, dermal matrix abnormalities, and solar elastosis. Clinical improvement of solar lentigines, scars, including keloids and hypertrophic scars, and photoaging have all been observed. Orringer et al have reported increases in type I procollagen messenger RNA and subsequent dermal matrix remodeling following one treatment with a pulsed dye laser. Whether this is secondary to thermal alterations of cellular milieu or to vascular-injury-induced cytokines, the result is dermal remodeling, reversal of photoaging, and partial rhytid correction.

The first laser designed to exploit the principle of selective photothermolysis was the flashlamp-pumped pulsed dye laser (PDL). The laser was optimized to treat port-wine stains. As the understanding of treatment of vascular lesions has progressed, so has the configuration of the PDL, in both composition of the dye (rhodamine) and

A

Type I Photorejuvenation
Indications

- **Vascular lesions, including:**
  - **Symptoms of rosacea, redness, flushing**
  - **Telangiectasias**
  - **Erythema post laser resurfacing**

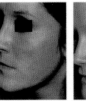
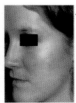

B

Type I Photorejuvenation
Indications

- **Pilosebaceous changes**
- **Decreased pore size**
- **Skin smoothing**

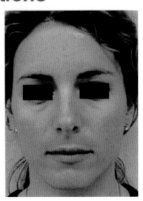

C

Type I Photorejuvenation
Indications

- **Pigmentary skin changes, including**
  - **Pigmentary sun damage**
  - **Mottled pigmentation**
  - **Hyperpigmentation**
  - **Photoaging**
  - **Lentigines**
  - **Dyschromia**
  - **Post peel or post ablative techniques: lines of demarcation**

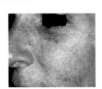
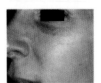

Figure 5.2 (A–C):Type I photoaging indications. *Republished with permission. Sadick NS 2003 Update on non-ablative light therapy for rejuvenation: a review. Lasers in Surgery and Medicine 32:120-128.*

Type II Photorejuvenation

- **Dermal and Subcutaneous Senescence**
  - **Rhytides**
  - **Lipodystrophy**

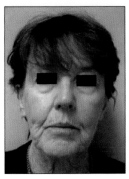

Figure 5.3 Type II Photoaging indications. *Republished with permission. Sadick NS 2003 Update on non-ablative light therapy for rejuvenation: a review. Lasers in Surgery and Medicine 32:120-128.*

Box 5.2
Relative contraindications for non-ablative resurfacing

- Active dermatitis (i.e. acne, autoimmune disease, etc.)
- Active infection (i.e. herpes, impetigo, etc.)
- History of keloid/hypertrophic scar formation
- History of koebnerizing dermatitis (i.e. psoriasis, vitiligo, etc.)
- History of photoinduced dermatitis (i.e. polymorphous light eruption, lupus, etc.)
- History of oral retinoid use in the past 6–24 months
- Recent ablative resurfacing procedure
- Recent medium or deep chemical peel
- Recent surgery or treatment area requiring undermining

---

wavelength. In its approximate 30-year existence, the PDL has moved beyond its original 577 nm wavelength, which corresponds to a hemoglobin absorption peak, and its original 0.45 millisecond pulse duration. Now, commercially available PDLs emit wavelengths between 585 nm and 595 nm, which penetrate deeper into the dermis and into deeper vessels. Newer PDLs have greater pulse duration ranges, most generating pulse trains of up to 40 milliseconds, which avoid intravascular thrombosis in very small vessels and subsequent purpura. Other than direct vascular heating and a resulting increase in dermal temperature, vessel targeting can also create an inflammatory cascade that results in new collagen formation. Bjerring showed a 148% increase in type II collagen 2 weeks after low-fluence PDL treatment and only a 32% increase with IPL; however, the authors conceded that the IPL settings (4–7 J/cm^2) were lower than those used in conventional application for red- brown dyschromias.

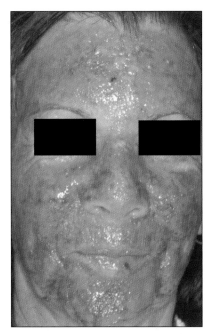

Figure 5.4 Photosensitivity reaction following photodynamic therapy. The patient is shown 6 days after photodynamic therapy. Reaction resolved after 3 weeks.

Table 5.2 Commonly used visible light / vascular lasers in non-ablative resurfacing*

Wavelength (nm)	Laser type	Energy	Pulse duration
532	Flash/arc lamp pumped KTP	Up to 950 J/cm²	5–100 ms
532	Diode-pumped KTP	0.1–5 W	5–1000 ms
585–595	Pulsed dye	Up to 40 J/cm²	0.45–40 ms, 350 ms
755	Alexandrite	1–50 J/cm²	0.5–300 ms
808	Diode	Up to 170 J/cm²	Up to 1000 ms
940	Diode	Up to 900 J/cm²	5–625 ms
532/1064	Q-switched Nd:YAG	Up to 16 J/cm²/Up to 37 J/cm²	5–20 ms
1064	Nd:YAG	Up to 990 J/cm², 120 J	0.1–300 ms

KTP = potassium titanyl phosphate; Nd:YAG = neodymium:yttrium-aluminum-garnet.
*This table represents a wide range of available lasers with some utility in non-ablative resurfacing. As each device has unique properties and settings, please refer to each specific device's manual for exact information to optimize patient treatment.

Other wavelengths that target hemoglobin in blood vessels have been shown to rejuvenate skin. The long-pulsed 755 nm alexandrite laser (Case study 1), the 810 nm diode, and the 1064 Nd:YAG lasers are used for deeper and larger-caliber vessels. The subsequent 'coincidental' dermal remodeling correlates to the depth of penetration of each respective laser. Weng et al have demonstrated that collagen synthesis by fibroblasts and antioxidant enzymes were significantly increased following irradiation with the 532 nm, 1064 nm Q-switched Nd:YAG, and 1064 nm long-pulse Nd:YAG lasers. The 1064 nm Nd:YAG laser induces deeper remodeling than the 532 nm laser due to its lower degree of dermal scattering and chromophore absorption at 1064 nm. Thus, some physicians use multiple lasers, such as the 532 nm laser to treat dyschromia and telangiectasia, and following it with a pass with the 1064 nm laser to obtain some deeper remodeling in the same treatment session.

CASE STUDY 1

A Caucasian female in her early 60s presents for total facial rejuvenation with request to focus on lentigenes, telangiectasias, and overall facial rejuvenation (Fig. 5.5A). The long-pulsed alexandrite 755 nm laser was used at a fluence of 36 J/cm² using an 8 mm spot size and a 3 ms pulse duration to treat the patient's forehead, cheeks, nose, and chin. At 6 weeks following her treatment, significant improvement in hyperpigmented macules, telangiectasias, and an overall more youthful appearance is appreciated (Fig. 5.5B).

Pearl 1

Combination treatment results in improved treatment results. The authors note improved outcomes with patients treated with combination using the 532 nm and 1064 nm lasers during the same treatment session. By using combination treatment, multiple chromophores can be targeted, with the 532 nm laser treating lentigines and telangiectasias, while the 1064 nm laser, by nature of its absorption spectrum, augments the rhytid correction of the 532 nm laser.

Near-infrared lasers have been used in a motion technique for skin rejuvenation. In one scenario, a 1064 nm laser equipped with a 5:7 mm spot size is deployed in a rapid back-and-forth fashion at 5 Hz and 12–15 J/cm². The device is moved from region to region based on either the surface temperature or when the heat becomes too uncomfortable to the unanesthetized patient. Typically, one achieves a surface temperature of about 39–42°C and then moves to an adjacent region. The lack of anesthetic is imperative in this approach, as excessive pain must be reported by the patient and should alert the operator to

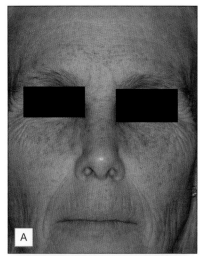

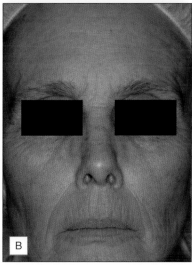

Figure 5.5 Patient treated with long-pulsed alexandrite laser for photorejuvenation: (**A**) pre-treatment, and (**B**) post-treatment.

move and prevent epidermal injury. The procedure (Laser Genesis, Cutera, Brisbane, CA) is easy to perform and results in only mild erythema postoperatively. In a study of 50 Asian patients evaluated by photography and biopsies, improvement in wrinkles, pore size, and elastin production were noted. No epidermal cooling was required. Another tool for NAR is the Q switched Nd YAG laser. Used in a motion technique at 5–10 Hz and 2–4 J/cm², the laser is applied with a 4–6 mm spot and multiple passes. Endpoints are mild erythema and the laser can be applied in multiple sessions 2–4 weeks apart. Often modest reduction in fine lines, scars, and dyschromia is observed.

Other devices that heat the mid-dermis include halogen lamps and xenon flashlamps. The output of the former ranges from 1100 to 1300 nm, and the output of the latter ranges from about 600 to 1200 nm. Like their laser near-infrared counterparts, the effect is gentle heating of the mid-dermis and upper hypodermis. These devices

straddle the applications of skin tightening and skin rejuvenation, which is a somewhat arbitrary distinction where tightening has been defined as overall skin contour enhancement. In contrast, these devices heat superficially enough that more general and ambiguous changes are observed. In one side-by-side study, a halogen lamp device improved skin laxity in 41% of patients. As in most of these types of studies, where gentle sustained heating is applied, the subjective improvement rates exceed objective outcome measures of improvement.

Adverse effects associated with all vascular lasers range from dyschromia, purpura, and blistering to scarring. Epidermal cooling techniques decrease epidermal heating and minimize pigmentary alteration. This addition is imperative in patients with Fitzpatrick IV–VI type skin treated with visible light lasers. Patients with a recent tan may also warrant a test spot. Epidermal cooling may be utilized prior to or following laser treatment by application of multiple different cooling devices, like a cold aluminum 'roller', ice packs, chilled sapphire windows, other contact cooling mechanisms, chilled air cooling or cryogen spray cooling. Purpura, blistering, and scarring can be avoided by knowledge and appropriate alteration of the fluence, spot size, and pulse duration when treating different skin types.

Pearl 2

When treating with modalities that utilize cooling mechanisms, it is important to minimize the condensation that can sometimes accumulate, which occurs most commonly with sapphire or glass windows. This condensation attenuates the laser beam and decreases the efficacy of the treatment.

Mid-infrared lasers (Table 5.3)

Clinical and histological evidence of non-ablative skin rejuvenation has been observed after use of mid-infrared lasers. The 1320 nm Nd:YAG laser was the first commonly used non-ablative mid-infrared laser to rejuvenate skin. When combined with surface cooling, collagen remodeling is achieved without epidermal damage. With water as the chromophore, the non-specific dermal thermal injury creates edema, vascular changes, and alterations in fibroblast assembly of dermal matrix constituents. The healing sequence can result in mild rhytid correction. The 1450 nm diode laser has been used for non-ablative rejuvenation in the same way as the 1320 nm Nd:YAG.

The 1540 nm erbium:glass laser similarly induces tissue water heating, thermal injury, and neocollagenesis. This laser penetrates to a depth intermediate between 1320 nm (deepest) and 1450 nm (shallowest) among this wavelength range. In planning strategies with all the mid-infrared wavelengths, the depth of penetration should coincide with the depth of solar elastosis.

Each of the non-fractional mid-infrared lasers uses a cooling system to minimize epidermal damage and pigmentary alteration. The 1320 nm Nd:YAG uses either a

Table 5.3 Commonly used mid-infrared lasers / devices in non-ablative resurfacing*

Wavelength (nm)	Laser type	Energy	Pulse duration (ms)	Spot sizes (mm)	Cooling
1319	Nd:YAG	Up to 30 J/cm²	5–200	6, 30 × 30	Integrated cooling
1320	Nd:YAG	5–40 J/cm²	30–200	6, 10	Integrated contact cooling, integrated cryogen spray
1450	Diode	Up to 25 J/cm²	210, 250	4–6	Integrated dynamic cooling device, integrated cryogen spray
1470	Diode	12 W	5–1000	Up to 15	None
1540	Erbium:glass	10–30 J/cm²	3–100	4	Sapphire lens
515–1200	Intense pulsed light	Up to 70 J/cm²	1–500 (single mode) 2.2–12.5 (pulsed mode)	10, 12, 15, 15 × 8, 15 × 10, 20 × 10, 20 × 30, 30 × 10, 34 × 8, 35 × 15, 34 × 18, 50 × 25, 50 × 10, 46 × 18, 46 × 10	Chilled tip contact cooling

Nd:YAG = neodymium:yttrium-aluminum-garnet.
*This table represents a wide range of available lasers with some utility in non-ablative resurfacing. As each device has unique properties and settings, please refer to each specific device's manual for exact information to optimize patient treatment.

pre- or post-laser spray, while the 1450 nm diode laser applies cryogen before, during, and after the laser pulse. These combinations of longer wavelengths and surface cooling make these lasers favorable for Fitzpatrick IV, V, and VI skin types. However, particularly in the case of the 1450 nm system, where the total spray time is delivered over a long period (up to 220 ms), there is a risk of cryoinjury. The shorter spray times with the 1320 nm laser and the 5°C sapphire lens incorporated into the 1540 nm erbium:glass laser have not been associated with cryoinjury.

The side effect profile of each of these lasers has a direct correlation with the fluences applied in the treatment of rhytides or acne scars. Although the efficacy of these devices has proven modest in most cases, providers must be cautious to avoid pigmentary changes and the rare case of scarring, which is typically secondary to treating using a fluence that is too high.

Pearl 3

Caution must be used when using higher fluences in smaller cosmetic units (i.e. upper lip). High fluences may increase bulk heating and increase risk for hyperpigmentation or scarring.

Intense pulsed light

IPL devices emit a broad spectrum of wavelengths between 400 and 1200 nm to target multiple structures. These devices, although not emitting monochromatic, collimated, or coherent light, still use selective photothermolysis. IPL can be used to target specific chromophores while avoiding others by using available filters to select certain wavelengths within the 400–1200 nm range. Shorter wavelengths can be used to treat lighter-skinned patients or the spectrum can be 'red shifted' through filters or through electronic modulation to minimize melanin absorption in darker-skinned patients. Peaks of hemoglobin absorption can be selectively used to target vascular structures. Finally, for purposes of non-ablative skin rejuvenation, dermal water can be targeted to induce photothermal initiation of neocollagenesis.

The utility and potential risks of the IPL are associated with its diversity. An IPL can be configured to treat the most clinically relevant chromophores (water, melanin, hemoglobin), and thereby multiple dermatologic conditions. There are many available IPL units with a wide array of designs and treatment parameters. Even though newer systems have improved user friendly pre-programmed settings, one should become comfortable with one or two IPL systems as each has different interfaces, wavelength spectrums, filters, power outputs, pulse profiles, cooling systems, and spot sizes. Some of the parameter sets do not allow different IPL systems to be compared easily. For example, there are some IPL devices that calculate their fluences based partly on theoretical modeling and photon recycling whereas others determine fluence based solely on an actual output at the sapphire or quartz window on the handpiece tip. Thus, moving from one IPL device to another does not mean that you will get the same outcome with the same settings on the display panel. A spectrophotometer (color meter) is provided with one new IPL (Icon, Palomar Medical Technologies, Burlington, MA). The meter transmits the patient pigment level directly to the IPL via Bluetooth™ technology. The graphic user interface then shows suggested test spot settings for that particular skin region.

Pearl 4

Good contact between the handpiece and the skin along with taut pressure may maximize the depth of the laser penetration, evenly treat the skin within the spot size, and will decrease the risk of postinflammatory hyperpigmentation. When using IPL devices to treat the face, this becomes very important, especially in darker-pigmented skin, as the face is full of many crevices and contours and most IPL devices utilize a rectangular handpiece, which makes good contact difficult in the perinasal and periocular regions.

Finally, although the utility of IPL devices allows for treatment of a wide variety of conditions, the addition of radiofrequency has been utilized to supplement and improve outcomes with use of IPL devices (Elos, Syneron). Bipolar radiofrequency exhibits a preference for warmer tissue. This technology takes this property into consideration by utilizing the IPL system to heat the target chromophore and then using the radiofrequency technology to target the now 'warmer' tissue target. Contact cooling helps avoid epidermal damage and keep the tissue heat in the dermis. This synergistic technology has proven efficacy in treatment of photoaging, helping reduce wrinkles, lentigenes, and telangiectasias.

Light-emitting diodes

LEDs for photoaging consist of a panel(s) of numerous small lamps that emit low-intensity light. Some companies have miniaturized these devices to handheld units that are used at home, while most professionals are using panels that can treat the entire face in one treatment session. One advantage of LED devices is that they are well tolerated by patients. With no pain, large surface areas of skin can be treated simultaneously.

Typically, LED devices emit a range of wavelengths. These devices are available in various wavelengths from blue to infrared. Depending on the wavelength and treatment parameters, LEDs emit milliwatt light in a small range around a peak wavelength. Thus, for example, if one were to select a LED with a dominant wavelength of 500 nm, the device will likely emit light from approximately 480 to 520 nm.

The interaction of LED devices with the skin are unclear, though most believe that photomodulation of cell receptors, cell organelles, or existing protein products is partially responsible. Unlike many of the devices discussed above, non-thermal interactions with the extracellular matrix and fibroblasts remodel existing collagen, increase collagen production by fibroblasts, inhibit collagenase activity, and result in rhytid reduction.

One of the most popular LED systems is the Gentle Waves® device (Light BioScience, LLC, Virginia Beach, VA). The system generates 588 nm yellow light pulses with an on-time of 250 ms and off-times of 10 ms for a total of 100 pulses resulting in a total light dose of 0.1 J/cm². Although some trials showed significant improvement in pore size, skin tone, and texture, the most comprehensive controlled clinical trial showed no significant skin changes in objective outcomes after a series of treatments. Boulos found that there was a strong placebo effect with the 588 nm Gentle Waves® system, and that little objective improvement was observed by blinded raters. Despite the subjective improvement in two trials, objective improvement in blinded studies is unproven.

In a study of 633 nm and 830 nm LED biostimulation, two treatments per week over 4 weeks showed increases in collagen production and mild wrinkle improvement. In a study using a reconstructed skin substitute irradiated with 633 nm LED panels, increases in collagen production were also observed. Additionally, in the clinical arm of the study, patients receiving treatment 3 times a week for 4 weeks (12 treatments) were found to get mild to moderate wrinkle improvement compared with sham treatment.

Photodynamic therapy

Over the past 20 years, photosensitizing agents have enjoyed an increasing role in medical and cosmetic dermatology. Twenty percent 5-aminolevulenic acid (5-ALA, a 'prodrug') is absorbed by rapidly proliferating epidermal and dermal cells and converted into photoreactive products of the hemoglobin pathway, most notably protoporphyrin IX (see Fig. 5.1). Protoporphyrin IX is subsequently activated by certain wavelengths of light, as highlighted by the absorption peaks in Figure 5.1, resulting in singlet oxygen production and resultant cellular destruction.

Many light sources have been used for PDT (Box 5.3). This variety is possible owing to multiple absorption peaks by protoporphyrin IX. The largest peaks are at 417, 540, 570, and 630 nm. The PDL, IPL, and LED devices have all been used to activate protoporphyrin IX. There are many variables that affect the immediate PDT response, among them the ALA incubation time, pre-ALA skin preparation regimen, degree of skin photodamage, anatomical region, light dose, wavelength range, and power density. Overall, lower power densities (i.e. continuous wave light sources) create more singlet oxygen than pulsed light. Also, we have found that applying numbing creams simultaneously with the ALA solution can accelerate ALA absorption and thereby accelerate protoporphyrin formation, leading to a much more robust response.

Pearl 5

Microdermabrasion, chemical peels, acetone, alcohol, retinoids, and thorough cleansing of the treatment area have all been advocated for making the stratum corneum more uniform, increasing the likelihood that the PDT will penetrate deeper and more evenly.

Many studies have shown the improvement of actinic keratoses and acne with PDT. Some studies have shown evidence of increased collagen formation. Gold et al have reported improvement in crow's feet, skin texture,

Box 5.3
Lasers and light sources used with ALA-PDT

1. **IPL Quantum SR* (Lumenis Ltd., Yokneam, Israel)**
   a. 560 nm filter
   b. double pulse (2.4/4.0 msec with 10 msec delay)
   c. single pass with no overlap
   d. 25 to 35 J/cm²
2. **Lumenis One* (Lumenis Ltd., Yokneam, Israel)**
   a. 560 nm filter
   b. double pulse (4.0/4/0 msec with 20 msec delay)
   c. single pass with no overlap
   d. 15 to 25 J/cm²
3. **VascuLight SR* (Lumenis Ltd., Yokneam, Israel)**
   a. 560 nm filter
   b. double pulse (3.0/6.0 msec with 10 msec delay)
   c. single pass with no overlap
   d. 30 to 35 J/cm²
4. **EsteLux Pulsed Light System* (Palomar Medical Technologies, Burlington, MA)**
   a. 20 msec
   b. 19 to 30 J/cm²
   c. single pass with no overlap
5. **Photogenica V Star* (Cynosure Inc., Chelmsford, MA)**
   a. 585 nm or 595 mn wavelength PDL
   b. 10 mm spot size
   c. 40 msec pulse width
   d. 7.5 J/cm²
   e. 2 passes with 50% overlap
6. **V Beam (Candela Corp., Wayland, MA)**
   a. 595 nm PDL
   b. 10 mm spot size
   c. 6 msec pulse width
   d. 7.5 J/cm²
   e. 2 passes with 50% overlap
7. **ClearLight* (Lumenis Ltd., Yokneam, Israel)**
   a. 405 nm to 420 nm blue light
   b. 8 to 10 minutes under light
8. **BluU* (Dusa Pharmaceuticals, Wilmington, MA)**
   a. 417 nm +/– 5 nm blue light
   b. 8 to 15 minutes under light
9. **SkinStation* (Radiancy, Orangeburg, NY)**
   a. 500 to 1200 nm pulsed light
   b. 2 passes
   c. 45 J/cm²
10. **Aurora (Syneron Medical Ltd., Yokneam, Israel)**
    a. 580 nm to 980 nm
    b. optical energy of 16–22 J/cm²
    c. single pass
11. **PhotoLight* (Cynosure Inc., Chelmsford, MA)**
    a. 550 nm filter
    b. 8 J/cm²
    c. 15 to 20 msec
    d. single pass
12. **Sciton BBL* (Sciton Inc., Palo Alto, CA)**
    a. 560 nm BBL filter
    b. 14 J/cm²
    c. 12 msec
    d. single pass

The following lasers and light secretes are correctly being used by the author for ALA-PDT treatments for aces regards (other devices listed above also able to be used) with similar parameters as listed above:

1. ClearLight
2. BluU
3. IPL Quantum
4. Lumenis One
5. VascuLight SR
6. SkinStation

Data from Gold MH 2005 Skin and Aging 13(2):Feb.
*Device used by author: other settings from colleagues.
(Reproduced with permission of the publisher. Chart appeared in *Skin & Aging 13(2):49, 2005.*)

mottled hyperpigmentation, telangiectasias, and actinic keratosis with the addition of 5-ALA prior to IPL treatment (Case study 2).

CASE STUDY 2

A 57-year-old white male presents for evaluation and treatment of overall actinic damage, including actinic keratoses and lentigenes on his cheeks (Fig. 5.6A). Treatment was initiated by the application of Levulan® (DUSA Pharmaceuticals, Inc), a 2-hour incubation period, and blue light for 5 minutes; 5% lidocaine cream was placed on the treated areas for the last 30 minutes of the patient's ALA incubation, which has been shown to enhance ALA absorption and photodynamic therapy effect. Finally, the 532 nm long-pulsed green laser (Gemini®, Laserscope, San Jose, CA) was used with cooling at a fluence of 7 J/cm² at 18 ms using a 10 mm spot size to treat the entire cheek and nose area. Two months after treatment, the patient's actinic damage was significantly improved (Fig. 5.6B).

Overview of treatment strategy

Patient selection is important to obtain the best expectation–outcome match. Patients may present for treatment of wrinkles and not the other characteristics of photoaging, even though telangiectasia or lentigines may be present. The modality of treatment is also important as each light device offers unique advantages. For example, if the patient presents with a concern of excessive telangiectasia, use of the 532 nm potassium titanyl phosphate (KTP), a PDL, or an IPL device may be warranted. If the goal is to obtain deeper dermal remodeling, one could consider longer-wavelength modalities such as the mid-infrared devices. Due to the widespread use and versatility of IPLs, many dermatologists are treating multiple photoaging characteristics simultaneously, including hyperpigmentation, telangiectasia, rhytides, and skin texture abnormalities. If the patient presents with actinic keratoses, PDT can be performed either at the same appointment or before or after visible pulsed light treatment for

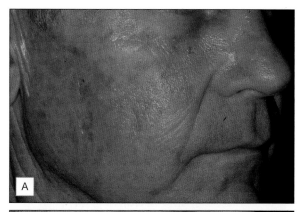

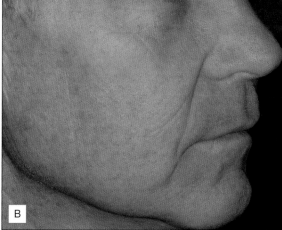

Figure 5.6 Treatment of photoaging with ALA/Gemini 532 nm long-pulsed green laser: (A) pre-treatment, and (B) post-treatment.

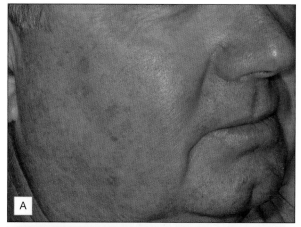

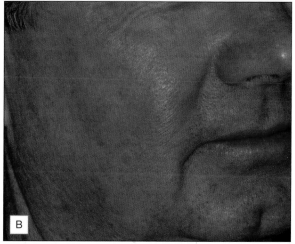

Figure 5.7 Patient treated with combination therapy ALA/PDT and pulsed dye laser with marked improvement in actinic damage, lentigines, telangiectasias, and overall skin quality: (A) pre-treatment, and (B) post-treatment.

red and brown dyschromias. Often a patient presents with multiple telangiectasias and actinic keratoses. If one uses only a vascular laser or IPL, the actinic damage and the associated telangiectasias within the actinic keratoses will persist or relapse; accordingly, either pre-treatment with 5% fluorouracil cream or PDT will enhance the total rejuvenation effect and decrease the likelihood of an incomplete response (Case study 3).

CASE STUDY 3

A 51-year-old white male presents with hyperpigmented patches along bilateral cheeks as well as multiple actinic keratoses on his cheeks and forehead (Fig. 5.7A). Treatment was initiated by the application of Levulan® (DUSA Pharmaceuticals, Inc.), a 2-hour incubation period, and photodynamic therapy illumination. He was subsequently treated with the V-Beam Perfecta® (Candela Corporation, Wayland, MA) using a 10 mm spot size, 8 J/cm², a 10 ms pulse duration, with 3 bars of cooling to bilateral cheeks. At 6-week follow-up, there was significant reduction in actinic keratoses, solar lentigenes, telangiectasias, and overall facial rejuvenation (Fig. 5.7B).

With all lasers or light modalities, preparation of the patient and the clinical setting are important. All required items (gauze, gel, eye protection, etc.) should be placed on an easily accessible Mayo stand. The treating handpiece should be cleaned according to the manufacturer's instructions and the device be positioned so that no cords or fibers are under tension.

Many physicians advocate pre-treatment preparatory use of a topical retinoid, not only to maximize medical photo-correction, but also to reduce the risk of dyspigmentation following treatment. Just prior to the procedure, the patient's skin should be cleansed. Any residual debris, including oil, make-up, lotions, or topical anesthetics (if administered), may impede the delivery of light to the skin. Some practitioners use alcohol pads to wipe off any residual after the bulk of the debris is removed. This should be allowed to completely dry prior to treatment.

The physician should always obtain pre-treatment photographs. The patient should be placed and draped in a position that allows full access to the treatment area. This is typically achieved by placing the patient in the supine position to treat photodamaged areas such as the face, neck, chest, and forearms. Appropriate goggles or eye shields (internal or external depending on the treatment area) are then applied to assure proper ocular protection. It is helpful to inform the patient who has appropriate eye protection about the likelihood of seeing a flash of light during the procedure. Many patients become anxious regarding the dangers of lasers when they see a flash of light even when they have goggles or shields over their eyes. Informing them that they are adequately protected, even when they see a flash of light adjacent to the shields, puts them at ease.

Conclusion

Non-ablative rejuvenation remodels photodamaged dermal constituents without inducing an epidermal wound. Minimal recovery times make this approach appealing to physicians and patients alike. Reversal of dyschromias (pigment and vascular) are reasonably predictable. Unfortunately, at this point, in the eyes of many clinicians, objective clinical and histologic outcomes with nonablative technologies do not correlate with clinician expectations, with the exception of novel fractional lasers and visible light technologies that target pigmented and vascular lesions.

Further Reading

Alam M, Dover JS 2004 Treatment of photoaging with topical aminolevulinic acid and light. Skin Therapy Letter 9(10):7-9

Barolet D, Roberge CJ, Auger FA, et al 2009 Regulation of skin collagen metabolism in vitro using a pulsed 660 nm LED light source: clinical correlation with a single-blinded study. Journal of Investigative Dermatology 129(12):2751-2759

Berlin AL, Hussain M, Goldberg DJ 2007 Cutaneous photoaging treated with a combined 595/1064 nm laser. Journal of Cosmetic and Laser Therapy 9(4):214-217

Bhat J, Birch J, Whitehurst C, et al 2005 A single-blinded randomised controlled study to determine the efficacy of Omnilux Revive facial treatment in skin rejuvenation. Lasers in Medical Science 20(1):6-10

Boulos PR, Kelley JM, Falcao MF, et al 2009 In the eye of the beholder – skin rejuvenation using a light-emitting diode photomodulation device. Dermatologic Surgery 35(2):229-239

Chan HH, Yu CS, Shek S, et al 2008 A prospective, split face, single-blinded study looking at the use of an infrared device with contact cooling in the treatment of skin laxity in Asians. Lasers in Surgery and Medicine 40(2):146-152

Cho SB, Lee SJ, Kang JM, et al 2010 Treatment of refractory arcuate hyperpigmentation using a fractional photothermolysis system. Journal of Dermatologic Treatment 21(2):107-108

Dang Y, Ren Q, Hoecker S, et al 2005 Biophysical, histological and biochemical changes after non-ablative treatments with the 595 and 1320 nm lasers: a comparative study. Photodermatology, Photoimmunology and Photomedicine 21(4):204-209

Dang Y, Ren Q, Li W, et al 2006 Comparison of biophysical properties of skin measured by using non-invasive techniques in the KM mice using 595 nm pulsed dye, 1064 nm Q-Switched Nd:YAG and 1320 nm Nd:YAG laser non-ablative rejuvenation. Skin Research and Technology 12(2):119-125

Goldman MP, Alster TS, Weiss R 2007 A randomized trial to determine the influence of laser therapy, monopolar radiofrequency treatment, and intense pulsed light therapy administered immediately after hyaluronic acid gel implantation. Dermatologic Surgery 33(5):535-542

Gu W, Liu W, Yang X, et al 2011 Effects of intense pulsed light and ultraviolet A on metalloproteinases and extracellular matrix expression in human skin. Photomedicine and Laser Surgery 29(2):97-103

Karrer S, Baumler W, Abels C, et al 1999 Long-pulse dye laser for photodynamic therapy: investigations in vitro and in vivo. Lasers in Surgery and Medicine 25(1):51-59

Katz BE, Truong S, Maiwald DC, et al 2007 Efficacy of microdermabrasion preceding ALA application in reducing the incubation time of ALA in laser PDT. Journal of Drugs in Dermatology 6(2):140-142

Kim HS, Yoo JY, Cho KH, et al 2005 Topical photodynamic therapy using intense pulsed light for treatment of actinic keratosis: clinical and histopathologic evaluation. Dermatologic Surgery 31(1):33-36; discussion 36-37

Kono T, Groff WF, Sakurai H, et al 2007 Comparison study of intense pulsed light versus a long-pulse pulsed dye laser in the treatment of facial skin rejuvenation. Annals of Plastic Surgery 59(5):479-483

Lee SY, Park KH, Choi JW, et al 2007 A prospective, randomized, placebo-controlled, double-blinded, and split-face clinical study on LED phototherapy for skin rejuvenation: clinical, profilometric, histologic, ultrastructural, and biochemical evaluations and comparison of three different treatment settings. Journal of Photochemistry and Photobiology B 88(1):51-67

Liu H, Dang Y, Wang Z, et al 2008 Laser induced collagen remodeling: a comparative study in vivo on mouse model. Lasers in Surgery and Medicine 40(1):13-19

Ross EV, Sajben FP, Hsia J, et al 2000 Nonablative skin remodeling: selective dermal heating with a mid-infrared laser and contact cooling combination. Lasers in Surgery and Medicine 26(2):186-195

Ross EV, Zelickson BD 2002 Biophysics of nonablative dermal remodeling. Seminars in Cutaneous Medicine and Surgery 21(4):251-265

Ruiz-Rodriguez R, Lopez-Rodriguez L 2006 Nonablative skin resurfacing: the role of PDT. Journal of Drugs in Dermatology 5(8):756-762

Sadick NS 2003 Update on non-ablative light therapy for rejuvenation: a review. Lasers in Surgery and Medicine 32(2):120-128

Sadick NS 2008 A study to determine the efficacy of a novel handheld light-emitting diode device in the treatment of photoaged skin. Journal of Cosmetic Dermatology 7(4):263-267

Seguchi K, Kawauchi S, Morimoto Y, et al 2002 Critical parameters in the cytotoxicity of photodynamic therapy using a pulsed laser. Lasers in Medical Science 17(4):265-271

Sterenborg HJ, van Gemert MJ 1996 Photodynamic therapy with pulsed light sources: a theoretical analysis. Physics in Medicine and Biology 41(5):835-849

Tanaka Y, Matsuo K, Yuzuriha S 2011 Objective assessment of skin rejuvenation using near-infrared 1064-nm neodymium:YAG laser in Asians. Clinical, Cosmetic and Investigational Dermatology 4:123-130

Wang R, Liu W, Gu W, Zhang P 2011 Intense pulsed light protects fibroblasts against the senescence induced by 8-methoxypsoralen plus ultraviolet-A irradiation. Photomedicine and Laser Surgery 29(10):685-690

Weiss RA, McDaniel DH, Geronemus RG, et al 2005 Clinical trial of a novel non-thermal LED array for reversal of photoaging: Clinical, histologic, and surface profilometric results. Lasers in Surgery and Medicine 36(2):85-91

Weiss RA, McDaniel DH, Geronemus RG, et al 2005 Clinical experience with light-emitting diode (LED) photomodulation. Dermatologic Surgery 31(9 pt 2):1199-1205

Weng Y, Dang Y, Ye X, et al 2011 Investigation of irradiation by different nonablative lasers on primary cultured skin fibroblasts. Clinical and Experimental Dermatology 36(6):655-660

Non-ablative fractional laser rejuvenation

6

Chung-Yin Stanley Chan, Andrei Metelitsa,
Jeffrey S. Dover

Summary and Key Features

- Non-ablative fractional resurfacing is a safe and effective treatment that has become the cornerstone for facial rejuvenation and acne scarring
- It is effective in treating a variety of conditions including acne scarring, mild to moderate photoaging, and some forms of dyspigmentation
- Non-ablative fractional photothermolysis (NAFR) has minimal downtime with almost no restrictions on activity immediately following treatment
- Common areas treated include the face, neck, chest, and hands
- All Fitzpatrick skin phototypes can be treated provided settings are adjusted accordingly
- The preoperative consultation is a vital component of the treatment regimen to ensure optimal outcomes
- Erythema and edema are common sequelae after treatment and resolve within a few days
- Long-term complications are exceedingly rare
- Technology in the field is changing rapidly and the selection of equipment is based on individual preference
- Home-based devices are a new frontier for lasers but will not replace office-based systems

Introduction

Treatment approaches are constantly being developed and refined in the field of skin rejuvenation. Since its original introduction in 2004, fractional photothermolysis has provided rejuvenation treatment approaches that are both effective and safe. Developed by Anderson & Manstein, fractional photothermolysis generates targeted microthermal treatment zones (MTZs), columns of thermally denatured skin of controlled width and depth, in the dermis. Their original device utilizing this technology induced necrosis within the epidermis and dermis while leaving the stratum corneum histologically intact and was thus termed non-ablative fractional photothermolysis (NAFR).

One of the main advantages of NAFR is limited discomfort and the minimal recovery that is required after the procedure. In contrast to conventional resurfacing devices, fractional photothermolysis treats only a fraction of this skin, allowing for rapid epidermal repair from undamaged areas. Although multiple treatment sessions are required to achieve the desired outcome, downtime is limited to an average of 3 days of redness and swelling as opposed to an average of 7–10 days of an open wound after aggressive non-fractional ablative resurfacing. Combined with an excellent safety profile, NAFR has become the cornerstone of laser skin rejuvenation for the treatment of photoaging and acne scarring and a variety of other clinical applications.

Pathophysiology

In fractional photothermolysis, a regular array of pixelated light energy creates focal areas of epidermal and dermal tissue damage or microthermal treatment zones (MTZ) (Fig. 6.1). Since its inception, several different lasers have been developed to take advantage of this technological advance. Each laser has parameters that can modify the density, depth, and size of the vertical columns of MTZs. The individual wounds created by FP are surrounded by healthy tissue resulting in a much quicker healing process when compared with traditional ablative skin resurfacing. This targeted damage with MTZ is hypothesized to stimulate neocollagenesis and collagen remodeling leading to the clinical improvements seen in scarring and photoaging. In the original study by Manstein et al., the histologic changes seen after NAFR were elegantly described. Immediately following treatment, lactate dehydrogenase (LDH) viability staining showed both epidermal and dermal cell necrosis within a sharply defined column correlating with the MTZ. There was continued loss of dermal cell viability 24 hours after treatment, but via a mechanism of keratinocyte migration, the epidermal defect had been repaired. One week after treatment, individual MTZs were still evident by LDH staining, but after 3 months there was no histologic evidence of loss of cell viability. Water serves as the target chromophore allowing for thermal damage to epidermal keratinocytes and collagen.

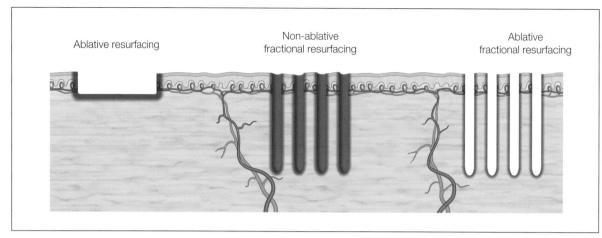

Figure 6.1 Diagram showing the differences between traditional ablative, non-ablative fractional, and ablative fractional resurfacing. With the fractional laser technology, microthermal treatment zones are created with intervening islands of unaffected tissue. Healing time is significantly less, and the energy can safely reach deeper into the dermis.

Hantash and colleagues demonstrated a unique mechanism of tissue repair with fractional photothermolysis. In 2006, they demonstrated, using an elastin antibody, that damaged dermal content was incorporated into columns of microscopic epidermal necrotic debris (MEND) and shuttled up through the epidermis and extruded in a process of transepidermal elimination. This mechanism, which had not been described with previous laser technologies, explains the elimination of altered collagen in photoaging and scars and was also hypothesized to provide novel treatment strategies for pigmentary disorders like melasma as well as depositional diseases like amyloid and mucinoses.

Epidemiology

According to the American Society for Plastic Surgery statistics, which provides a comprehensive estimate on the total number of cosmetic procedures performed in the United States, minimally invasive cosmetic procedures have increased by more than 100% since 2000. In 2010, over 300 000 non-ablative laser skin resurfacing procedures were performed with the majority done on females.

Equipment

As the technology of fractional photothermolysis continues to evolve, new devices continually come to market. A list of currently available NAFR systems is given in Table 6.1. The table is not comprehensive and, as one can imagine, the devices will change constantly. This section will provide a brief description of a few of the more commonly used devices.

The original non-ablative fractional resurfacing system described by Manstein featured a scanning handpiece with a 1500 nm wavelength. The updated, currently available model, the Fraxel re:store (Solta Medical, Hayward, CA),

employs a 1550 nm erbium glass laser. The device has tunable settings to adjust the density of the MTZs and energy depending on the treatment. Density can be varied to treat anywhere from 5 to 48% while energy settings can be adjusted to control depth of penetration from 300 to 1400 μm. Most of the studies available on non-ablative fractionated lasers are based on this device.

Solta Medical's newest addition, the Fraxel Dual, couples the 1550 nm erbium laser with a 1927 nm thulium fiber laser in one platform. The thulium laser provides a more superficial treatment option and better addresses dyspigmentation while the 1550 nm penetrates deeper to stimulate collagen remodeling. The system increases flexibility, allowing the practitioner to switch between the two lasers to tailor treatment accordingly. Parameters can be adjusted similarly to the Fraxel re:store. Cooling is also built in with the Fraxel Dual.

Palomar Medical Technologies (Burlington, MA) offers an intense pulsed light platform with individual handpieces that attach to a single unit to cover a wide range of uses. The Lux1440 and Lux1540 handpieces provide two wavelength options (1440 and 1550 nm) for fractional non-ablative photothermolysis. In addition, the company has developed a new XD Microlens for their non-ablative laser handpieces. In their study, the company claims that, as the dermis is compressed by the optical pins on the handpiece, the pins are brought closer to deeper targets and the interstitial water is displaced from the dermal–epidermal junction into the surrounding spaces. With less water to absorb, scattering of the laser light is reduced enabling increased absorption of the light by deeper targets.

The Affirm (Cynosure, Inc., Westford, MA) is a 1440 nm Nd:YAG laser device that utilizes a proprietary Combined Apex Pulse (CAP) technology. The technology creates columns of coagulated tissue surrounded by uncoagulated tissue columns, which purportedly improves

Table 6.1 Non-ablative fractional lasers

Device	Manufacturer	Type	Wavelength (nm)
Affirm	Cynosure (Westford, MA)	Nd:YAG	1440 +/– 1320
Clear+ Brilliant	Solta Medical (Hayward, CA)	Diode	1440
Fraxel re:fine	Solta Medical (Hayward, CA)	Erbium	1410
Fraxel re:store (former SR 1550)	Solta Medical (Hayward, CA)	Erbium	1550
Fraxel dual	Solta Medical (Hayward, CA)	Erbium + thulium	1550 + 1927
Lux 1440	Palomar Medical Technologies Inc. (Burlington, MA)	Nd:YAG	1440
Lux 1540	Palomar Medical Technologies Inc. (Burlington, MA)	Erbium	1540
Matrix RF	Syneron (Irvine, CA)	Diode + bipolar RF	915 + RF
Mosaic	Lutronic (San Jose, CA)	Erbium	1550
Sellas 1550	Enhanced Image Technologies (Charlotte, NC)	Erbium	1550

Box 6.1
Clinical indications for non-ablative fractional resurfacing

- Photoaging
- Scarring (atrophic, hypertrophic, hypopigmented)
- Disorders of pigmentation (melasma, nevus of Ota, drug-induced pigmentation)
- Poikiloderma of Civatte
- Premalignant conditions (actinic keratoses, disseminated superficial actinic porokeratosis)
- Striae distensae
- Vascular disorders (telangiectatic matting, residual hemangioma)

---

treatment efficacy. The Affirm uses a stamping handpiece with two spot sizes and energies that penetrate up to 300 μm in depth. A recent advance has been the addition of their multiplex technology, which stacks a 1320 nm wavelength with the 1440 nm system, allowing for penetration down to 1000–3000 μm.

Applications

While NAFR is currently approved by the US Food and Drug Administration for the treatment of benign epidermal pigmented lesions, periorbital rhytides, skin resurfacing, melasma, acne and surgical scars, actinic keratoses, and striae, it has been reported to be used in many other clinical settings (Box 6.1).

Photoaging

With their seminal study in 2004 using a prototype non-ablative fractional resurfacing device, Manstein and colleagues first demonstrated the clinical effectiveness of fractional photothermolysis by showing improvement in periorbital rhytides. Three months after four treatments with the fractionated device, 34% of patients had moderate to significant improvements and 47% had improvement in texture as rated by blinded investigators. Overall, 96% were noted to be 'better' post-treatment. The skin tightening seen after non-ablative fractional resurfacing is similar to ablative resurfacing with tightening within the first week after treatment, apparent relaxation at 1 month, and retightening at 3 months (Case study 1).

CASE STUDY 1
The right patient

A 58-year-old Caucasian male with mild rhytides and mild to moderate photodamage with scattered facial lentigines presents for consultation. You recommend a series of non-ablative fractional resurfacing laser procedures. Six months after the sixth laser procedure, you see the patient back in follow-up. He is delighted with his improvement in both texture and skin tone and subsequently refers a couple of his friends to see you.

The above patient is the ideal patient for non-ablative fractional resurfacing. These results are typical of the improvement we see in our patients when selected appropriately.

Subsequent reports have confirmed the efficacy of NAFR beyond just periorbital lines. Wanner and colleagues showed statistically significant improvement in photodamage of both facial and non-facial sites with 73% of patients improving at least 50%. In 2006, Geronemus also reported his experience with fractional photothermolysis, finding it to be effective in treating mild to moderate rhytides. Figures 6.2 and 6.3 show typical improvement in rhytides and pigmentation after treatment with non-ablative fractional resurfacing. For deeper rhytides, such as the vertical lines of the upper lip,

Figure 6.2 Improvement in moderate rhytides 1 month after two treatments with Fraxel 1927 nm. *(Photo courtesy of Solta Medical.)*

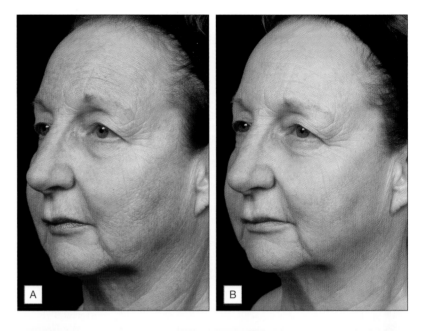

Figure 6.3 Improvement in rhytides and dyspigmentation 1 month after three treatments with Fraxel re:store. *(Photo courtesy of Solta Medical.)*

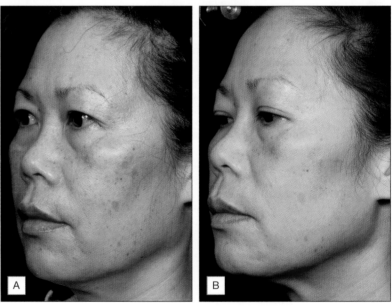

improvement is also seen but not nearly to the same degree as in ablative approaches.

NAFR is also considered to be an effective and safe treatment modality for photoaging off the face including the neck, chest, arms, hands (Fig. 6.4), legs, and feet. These body sites are typically very challenging to treat with other treatment modalities given either increased risks of complications (e.g. scarring) associated with ablative technologies or lack of efficacy that has been previously observed with other non-ablative devices. Jih et al reported statistically significant improvement in pigmentation, roughness, and wrinkling of the hands in ten patients treated with non-ablative fractional resurfacing. In our experience, we have found NAFR to be very safe when settings are adjusted accordingly.

Scarring

Scarring can induce a tremendous psychological, physical, and cosmetic impact on individuals. Previous therapeutic modalities in scar treatment include surgical punch grafting, subcision, dermabrasion, chemical peeling, dermal fillers, as well as laser resurfacing with ablative and non-ablative devices. Published studies have demonstrated

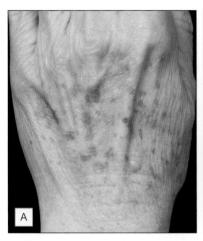

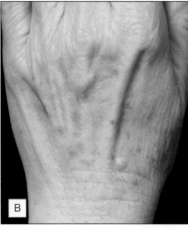

Figure 6.4 Improvement in rhytides and dyspigmentation of the hands 1 month after two treatments with Fraxel re:store. *(Photo courtesy of Solta Medical.)*

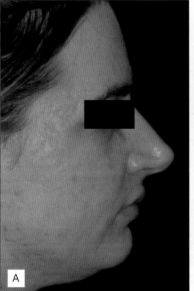

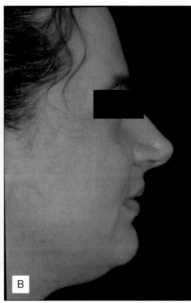

Figure 6.5 Significant improvement in texture and rolling acne scars 2 months after four treatments with Fraxel re:store.

that NAFR can be successfully utilized in the treatment of various forms of scarring, including acne scarring, with a very favorable safety profile (Fig. 6.5). Mechanistically, fractional photothermolysis allows controlled amounts of high energy to be delivered deep within the dermis resulting in collagenolysis and neocollagenesis, which smoothes the textural abnormalities of acne scarring. In a large clinical study, Weiss showed a median 50–75% improvement of acne scars using a 1540 nm fractionated laser system after three treatments at 4-week intervals with 85% of patients rating their skin as improved. Alster showed similarly impressive results in a study of 53 patients with mild to moderate acne scarring; 87% of patients who received three treatments at 4-week intervals showed at least 51–75% improvement in the appearance of their acne scars. Non-ablative fractional resurfacing, in our estimation, is the treatment of choice for facial acne scarring.

Pearl 1

Patients with deep acne scarring or severe rhytides often require high-energy settings, which correlates with deeper penetration of the laser and subsequent remodeling of collagen deeper in the cutis.

NAFR can also be safely used to treat acne scarring in darker-pigmented patients (Fig. 6.6). A study of 27 Korean patients with skin types IV or V that were treated with three to five non-ablative fractional resurfacing treatments revealed no significant adverse effects, specifically pigmentary alterations. Furthermore, all forms of acne scarring including ice-pick, boxcar, and rolling scars improved with eight patients (30%) reporting excellent improvement, 16 patients (59%) significant improvement, and three patients (11%) moderate improvement. With such

Figure 6.6 1 month after five treatments with Fraxel re:store showing significant improvement in acne scarring in a darkly pigmented patient. *(Photo courtesy of Solta Medical.)*

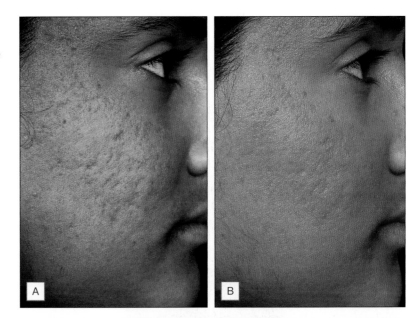

a good efficacy and safety profile, many clinicians prefer NAFR to ablative fractional photothermolysis when it comes to treating acne scarring.

NAFR can also be used in the treatment of other types of scars, including hypertrophic and hypopigmented scars. In a study of eight patients with hypertrophic scarring, all patients had improvement in their scars based on the physician's clinical assessment, with a mean improvement of 25–50%. While the flashlamp-pumped pulsed dye laser (PDL) had long been considered the laser of choice for treating hypertrophic scars, NAFR has showed tremendous promise when compared with PDL. In a study of 15 surgical scars in 12 patients, NAFR outperformed PDL in the improvement of surface pigmentation, texture change, and overall scar thickness. While more studies are needed, NAFR should be considered as a therapeutic option to be used in conjunction with or as an alternative to PDL.

Traditionally, treatment of hypopigmented scars has shown variable efficacy, but current evidence suggests that NAFR may be particularly useful. A pilot study of NAFR laser treatment showed a 51–75% improvement in hypopigmented scars in 6 of 7 patients treated. The mechanism of action for this repigmentation has been hypothesized to be secondary to migration of melanocytes from the pigmented, normal skin into the scar, resulting in blending of the border (Fig. 6.7).

Melasma

Despite individual reports documenting successful treatment of melasma with NAFR, long-term efficacy of such treatments is still uncertain. The first pilot study by Rokhsar & Fitzpatrick demonstrated an astounding 75–100% clearance of melasma in 60% of the patients at 3 months. Only one patient developed transient

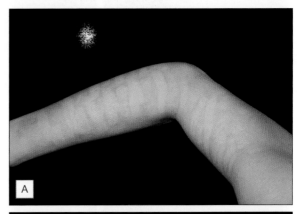

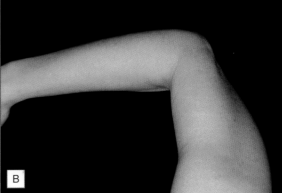

Figure 6.7 Improvement of hypopigmented scars 1 month after three treatments with Fraxel 1927 nm.

hyperpigmentation, which resolved. Another study by Goldberg et al. showed 'good' improvement of melasma in patients with skin type III. In this study, they also showed a decrease in melanocytes by electron microscopy. It has been proposed that dermal content, such as melanin, may be eliminated through the treatment channels through a mechanism termed melanin shuttling. However, other more recent studies have reported only modest improvement in melasma after treatment with NAFR. A study of 6 Chinese patients showed only a 35% mean improvement of melasma after three to four treatments. Finally, and perhaps most concerning, a recent study by Wind and associates showed worsening of hyperpigmentation following NAFR treatments in 9 out of 29 patients in a split-face randomized trial comparing laser to triple topical therapy. Not surprisingly, patient satisfaction was significantly lower on the laser-treated side.

> ## Pearl 2
>
> When treating dyschromia, which is generally more superficial, low energy levels with high-density settings should be used. The density of MTZs is higher at lower energy settings.

More recently, clinicians have been utilizing the 1927 thulium fiber laser for the treatment of melasma, but definitive studies are still lacking. In a pilot study by Polder & Bruce, a statistically significant 51% reduction in Melasma Area and Severity Index (MASI) Score was observed at 1 month after three to four laser treatments. The MASI score at 6 months, however, dropped to 34%. While initial NAFR reports showed promise in the treatment of melasma, it remains unclear how truly effective these lasers are in treating this chronic, stubborn condition and whether they alter the natural history of the condition. In our experience, NAFR has been useful in only a fraction of melasma patients.

Actinic keratoses

When treating actinic keratoses, treating the entire surface area of the affected anatomical site, known as field treating, is preferred to ensure that both clinically visible and microscopic lesions are covered. Initial attempts by Katz and associated to treat these precancerous lesions with fractional 1550 nm laser showed great clinical response with greater than 73% clearance 1 month post-treatment and 55.6% clearance at 6 months. Post-treatment biopsies, however, revealed histological persistence, and as a result, it has been recommended that NAFR not be used as a single treatment modality for actinic keratoses. More recently, fractional 1927 nm thulium laser was approved by the FDA for the treatment of actinic keratosis. Geronemus showed that, after a single treatment with the 1927 nm thulium laser, a mean of 63% of actinic keratoses were cleared and after two treatments, 84% of lesions cleared. Definitive data on histological clearance is still lacking. Although this early clinical data is exciting, and

our own clinical experience has been positive in treating extensive actinic keratoses on the limbs, it reminds us of the similar enthusiasm with NAFR in treating melasma. Further studies are needed, specifically ones with histological analysis, to prove its efficacy.

> ## Pearl 3
>
> The 1927 nm fractionated laser has a more superficial depth of penetration and is useful in treating actinic keratoses. It is especially useful in treating sun-induced lentigines of the face, neck, chest, and hands.

Striae

Although non-ablative fractional resurfacing has been FDA approved for the treatment of striae, only a few small studies have examined their effectiveness. Kim et al performed an early study demonstrating a substantial improvement in the appearance of striae distensae in six female subjects. Furthermore, histological examination showed an increase in epidermal thickness, collagen, and elastic fiber deposition. Other studies have also shown improvement, albeit modest, in striae appearance. One study showed good to excellent clinical improvement in 27% of patients, while another study showed a 26–50% improvement in 63% of patients. Further, large-scale studies need to be performed to more clearly define NAFR's effectiveness in treating striae. In our experience, the results, when appreciable, have been only modest. A recent consensus article recommends performing a large test area before having the patient commit to a series of treatments.

Poikiloderma of Civatte

Poikiloderma of Civatte is characterized by hyper- and hypopigmentation, atrophy, and telangiectasia. A case of one patient with poikiloderma of Civatte successfully treated with non-ablative fractional resurfacing has been reported. After a single treatment, there was noticeable improvement in pigmentation and texture. While pulsed dye lasers and intense pulse light sources are the treatments of choice for poikiloderma, fractional non-ablative devices are effective in improving overall color and texture in this condition.

Other conditions

NAFR has also been used to treat a host of other conditions including nevus of Ota, minocycline-induced hyperpigmentation, matted telangiectasias, residual fibrofatty tissue after hemangioma involution, recalcitrant disseminated superficial actinic porokeratosis, disseminated granuloma annulare, and colloid milium. Although difficult to gauge clinical response in single case reports, these reports provide evidence on the potential applications of this technology.

Patient selection

The preoperative consultation is crucial to maximize outcomes while minimizing complications. The clinician should assess the patient expectations and goals for treatment during this encounter. Showing patients before and after photos of a typical result can help set patient expectations regarding the efficacy of treatment. Even so, the patient must also understand that individual responses can vary.

Pearl 4

Take pre-treatment photos prior to treatment to document and assess response.

To achieve satisfactory results with NAFR, a series of four to six treatments is required. Typically these procedures are spaced out every 4 weeks and thus, an entire treatment regimen may take 6 months or more to complete (Case study 2). Those patients who prefer to have dramatic results after only one session are not the right candidates for non-ablative fractional resurfacing. Instead, these patients may benefit from fractional ablative resurfacing, which typically requires fewer treatment sessions, but has a much longer recovery. The procedure is painful, but topical anesthesia and forced-air cooling make the procedure tolerable in most. Redness and swelling last an average of 3 days.

CASE STUDY 2
Sometimes more is better

A 48-year-old male with severe rolling and box car acne scars has six non-ablative fractional resurfacing treatments with the 1550 nm device. Six months after the last treatment, he comes in wondering what else can be done for his acne scarring. On exam and comparison to pretreatment photos, you notice improvement in his acne scarring but also some room for further improvement. You recommend another two treatments and see him back 6 months after the 8th treatment. He is extremely pleased and says he noticed significantly more improvement from the final two treatments. This response is predictable as the improvement with non-ablative fractional resurfacing is curvilinear. The first two treatments yield very little visible improvement, the next two a bit more, and the final two show the greatest degree of change. Sometimes in patients with bad scarring we perform an additional two treatments but always wait 6 months to see the maximum improvement from the first six before deciding.

NAFR can be performed safely on patients with all Fitzpatrick skin types, but patients with darker skin types should be treated with caution. A study of fractional lasers in the treatment of acne scars by Alajlan & Alsuwaidan showed a high safety profile in those of ethnic skin. Although hyperpigmentation was noticed more commonly in darker skin patients, particularly when higher fluences

Box 6.2
Contraindications to non-ablative fractional resurfacing

- Pregnancy
- Lactation
- Active infection (bacterial, viral or fungal)
- Recent history of oral isotretinoin (less than 6 months prior)
- Patients with unrealistic expectations

were used, this effect was usually transient. To minimize complications in darker-skinned patients, bleaching creams along with lower treatment settings are recommended.

It is important to gather a history of prior laser procedures and responses, history of keloids, history of herpes simplex infection, skin phototype, history of postinflammatory hyperpigmentation (PIH), current medications including previous isotretinoin use, lidocaine allergy, pain tolerance, and anxiety level.

Patients who should not be treated with fractional resurfacing are women who are pregnant or lactating, those with active infection, particularly herpes simplex, and patients with a history of isotretinoin use in the past 6 months (Box 6.2). Furthermore, individuals with unrealistic expectations should not be treated.

The ideal patient for treatment is a fair skin (Fitzpatrick types I–III), motivated patient who desires attainable results with a few days downtime and has realistic expectations (Case study 3).

CASE STUDY 3
Just say no

A 76-year-old female comes for a preoperative consultation for non-ablative fractional resurfacing. She has been enjoying her summer on the beach and plans to return to her winter home in a few weeks. On exam, she has significant photodamage, sagging, and deep rhytides on a background of tanned skin with numerous lentigines. During the consultation, she makes it clear that since she is leaving soon, she wants to have one treatment that will improve her lines significantly with as little downtime as possible. She has read on the internet that non-ablative fractional resurfacing is a great treatment for her aging face with little recovery time and wants to know when she can start.

This patient is clearly not a suitable candidate for non-ablative fractional resurfacing. Patients should be counseled that, while NAFR is a highly effective treatment regimen with little downtime, a series of treatments spaced at least a couple of weeks apart is required to achieve those results. Additionally this patient who has a distinct tan would not be ideal for laser treatment as she would be at an increased risk for hyperpigmentation and more conservative treatment parameters would need to be used. Finally her sagging skin will not improve with this procedure. She might be a better candidate for ablative fractional resurfacing, non-surgical or surgical skin tightening.

Pretreatment

All patients should wear a broad-spectrum sunscreen (SPF >30) and should avoid sun exposure before, during and immediately after their treatments. There is no evidence that treating with topical hydroquinone for 1–2 months prior to non-ablative fractional resurfacing decreases the risk of postinflammatory pigmentation in individuals with darker skin types (type IV–VI). Nor is there any scientific proof that topical retinoids need to be discontinued prior to treatment in those with sensitive skin. In spite of this many physicians recommend using hydroquinone, and ask patients to discontinue retinoids, prior to non-ablative fractional resurfacing.

Pearl 5

Topical retinoids do not need to be discontinued prior to non-ablative fractional resurfacing. In some patients with sensitive skin doing so may make treatment more tolerable.

Pre-treatment with oral antiviral medications is recommended in those with a history of herpes simplex virus (HSV) infection (Box 6.3). Although some practitioners advocate the routine use of HSV prophylaxis regardless of previous infection, we do not feel that this is necessary. Firoz et al recently reported the first three cases of herpes zoster within the distribution of the trigeminal nerve after NAFR. The patients all had a history of chicken pox and none had received prophylaxis prior to treatment. Patients with a family history of herpes zoster and who have not had shingles themselves may thus benefit from the use antiviral treatment prior to treatment. Prophylactic antibiotics are not needed for non-ablative fractional resurfacing.

Box 6.3
Procedural steps in NAFR

1. Obtain consent and prepare patient:
   a. Review risks and limitations of procedure and answer questions
   b. Assess patient expectations
   c. Take pre-op photos
   d. Start prophylaxis for HSV if patient has a history of cold sores.
2. Wash the area to be treated.
3. Gently cleanse skin with alcohol wipe.
4. Apply topical anesthetic ointment and leave on for 1 hour prior to the procedure.
5. Perform procedure:
   a. Use a skin-cooling device
   b. Apply handpiece perpendicular to skin
   c. Take precaution not to bulk heat.
6. Prepare patient for discharge:
   a. Apply cold compresses or ice to minimize swelling
   b. Review post-treatment care
   c. Schedule follow-up appointment.

On the day of the first procedure, serial standardized photographs should be taken to allow patients to observe their treatment progress. Topical anesthesia should be applied 1 hour prior to starting the treatment. Several different anesthetic agents are currently available including 5% lidocaine, 7% lidocaine/7% tetracaine, 23% lidocaine/7% tetracaine, and 30% lidocaine. In our experience, anesthetic agents with tetracaine induce significant erythema leading to patient dissatisfaction. We use 30% lidocaine in our practice as it provides the most comfort with the least erythema. To minimize the risk of systemic toxicity from the topical anesthetics, areas no greater than 300–400 cm^2 should be treated during each session. Before the treatment, all of the anesthetic should be thoroughly washed off (Case study 4). Oral anxiolytics and analgesics may be required in a small fraction of patients who cannot tolerate the procedure with topical anesthesia alone. In those who find the procedure too uncomfortable with topical anesthesia, we first add ketorolac (Toradol®). In more anxious or intolerant individuals we have had success with diazepam and IM meperidine (Demerol®). IV sedation is not needed for this procedure. Metal eye protection is advised for the patient. All individuals in the treatment room should also wear eye protection. When it comes to selection of treatment parameters, a number of factors need to be considered including clinical indication, anatomical site, as well as skin phototype of the patients. In general, studies demonstrate that post-inflammatory pigmentation is less common when fractional resurfacing of darker skin is performed using lower density settings, fewer passes, and longer treatment intervals. Treatment of non-facial sites should be done with slightly lower density and fluence settings.

CASE STUDY 4
Toxicity

A 45-year-old, petite woman weighing 102 lbs presents for non-ablative fractional resurfacing of her face, neck, and chest to treat photoaging. She has not had treatment before and has some anxiety over the procedure. After counseling the patient and addressing her concerns, she gives her informed consent and pre-treatment photos are taken; 30% lidocaine gel is then applied over the face, neck, and chest.

Prior to her treatment, your schedule begins to run late and you are unable to start her treatment until an hour and a half after the topical anesthesia has been applied. She tolerates the first pass on her cheek but then suddenly becomes agitated and reports significant anxiety. Treatment is immediately stopped, but the woman begins to complain of nausea and perioral paresthesias. You start an infusion of normal saline and closely observe the patient over a couple of hours without further sequelae. Her serum lidocaine levels are elevated at 2 µg/ml.

To avoid this problem, topical anesthesia application should be limited to no more than 1 hour. Furthermore, large treatment areas should be avoided at one visit. A similar case has been reported in the literature (Marra 2006).

Pearl 6

Large treatment areas (>400 cm^2) should be avoided to reduce the risk of lidocaine toxicity.

Pearl 7

In darker-pigmented patients, treatment densities should be decreased; consider doing less passes in an effort to reduce the risk of hyperpigmentation.

General technique

We find the supine position most comfortable for the patient and practitioner. In this position, the practitioner can be seated comfortably with elbows close to 90° to alleviate fatigue and repetitive stress injury. During treatment, patient positioning is crucial to ensure perpendicular application of the laser handpiece. For example, when treating the neck, especially in the submandibular area, it is often helpful to have the chin tilted upward to allow for better exposure.

With the scanning handpiece of the Fraxel systems (Solta Medical, Hayward, CA), we deliver eight passes when treating acne scars, rhytides, and photoaging of the face. We use a double-pass, 50% overlap technique. One linear pass is delivered, the handpiece is brought to a complete stop, lifted, repositioned, and then returned along the same path for a second pass. The handpiece is then moved laterally by 50% and the technique is repeated until the treatment area is completed. As a result, each area is treated with four passes. For the next four passes, we direct the passes perpendicular to the first treatment to ensure complete and even laser coverage. Dividing the face into four quadrants also helps manage the treatment area and reduce the risk of overlap or missing a section.

For facial resurfacing, our settings are individualized according to patients' needs and tolerability. We often start with energy levels between 40–50 mJ and a treatment level of 6–8 (Table 6.2). The settings are often increased during subsequent visits if tolerated.

For stamping handpieces, the fractionated energy is delivered according to the tip size. For example with the StarLux system (Palomar Medical Technologies Inc., Burlington, MA) and the 15 mm Lux1540 handpiece, three to four passes are generally delivered with a 50% overlap in both directions. The handpiece should be lifted off the skin between each pulse, and pulse-stacking is not recommended. For facial resurfacing with the Lux1540 15 mm tip, we recommend using 10–15 mJ per microbeam with a pulse width of 10–15 ms. With the Affirm (Cynosure, Westford, MA) 1440 nm device, we use 3–5 mJ, depending on the tip size, and perform two passes for facial resurfacing, The number of passes and treatment parameters vary with the different machines and is beyond the scope of this chapter.

Cooling

A cooling device used in conjunction with the NAFR laser device should be standard for all treatments. A popular forced-air cooling device, the Zimmer Cryo (Zimmer Medizin Systems, Irvine, CA) increases patient comfort significantly. Some laser systems now also come with a built-in cooling device. In a study of 20 patients, 19 noted reduced pain with the addition of a cooling device.

Post-treatment

Upon completion of the treatment, patients are advised to ice their skin for several minutes and then periodically over the next few hours. Not only does this help with patient comfort, but it also reduces post-procedure swelling. Erythema develops immediately afterwards in all treated patients (Fig. 6.8) and typically resolves in 3 days. Use of non-comedogenic moisturizers is also recommended. Patients are advised to wear sun protection for several weeks after their treatment to reduce the risk of hyperpigmentation. In those with an increased risk of hyperpigmentation, hydroquinone may be started immediately after the procedure. We routinely wait to start lightening agents until we see the first signs of post-inflammatory pigmentation, which is usually around day 21 post-treatment. In a recent prospective study by Alster et al, a light emitting-diode device (Gentlewaves, Light BioSciences, Virginia Beach, VA) has been shown to decrease erythema intensity and duration following treatment, although the precise mechanism of action is unclear.

Safety and complications

NAFR is a well-tolerated procedure with an excellent safety profile. Fisher and Geronemus studied the immediate and short-term side effects showing a favorable side effect profile. In their study of 60 patients with skin types I–IV, all patients expectedly developed erythema immediately post-treatment, which in most patients resolved in 3 days. Xerosis occurred in 86.6% of patients, usually presenting 2 days after treatment and resolving by day 5 or 6. This was minimally bothersome and responded well to moisturization. Other frequently reported post-treatment side effects were transient and included facial edema (82%) and flaking (60%). Small, superficial scratches were also reported in 46.6% of patients. These scratches, which all resolve without sequelae, are thought to be related to tangential application of the hand piece or pulse stacking by inexperienced users. Pruritus (37%) and bronzing (26.6%) are also common side effects of treatment.

Perhaps the most valuable finding from this short-term study was the impact on the patient's quality of life; 72% reported limiting social activities by an average time of only 2.1 days, which is in stark contrast to the downtime seen with the conventional resurfacing laser. The most commonly attributed reasons were erythema and edema.

Table 6.2 Recommend treatment parameters

Device		Indication	Energy (mJ)	Pulse width (ms)	Treatment level*	Number of passes
1550 nm (Fraxel)		Facial resurfacing for most conditions other than melasma/dyspigmentation	40–70	–	6–10	8
		Non-facial resurfacing	20–40	–	6–10	–
		Melasma	10–20	–	4–6	8
1927 nm (Fraxel)		Facial resurfacing	10	–	5	8
		Non-facial resurfacing	10	–	3	8
		Melasma	5–10	–	2–4	8
1440 nm (StarLux/ Icon)	10 mm tip	Facial resurfacing	25–70	7–10	–	2
	15 mm tip	Facial resurfacing	6–10	7	–	1–3
1540 nm (StarLux/ Icon)	10 mm tip	Facial resurfacing	40–70	10–15	–	3–6
	15 mm tip	Facial resurfacing	10–15	10–15	–	3–4
	15 mm tip	Melasma†	5–12	10–15	–	2–5
1440 nm (Affirm)	10 mm tip	Facial resurfacing	3–5	–	–	2
	14 mm tip	Facial resurfacing	3–4	–	–	2

*Treatment level for darker skin types (IV–VI) should be decreased to reduce the risk of hyperpigmentation.
†For treating.

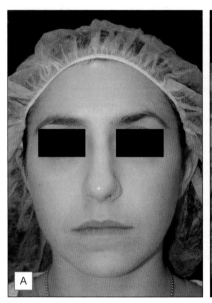 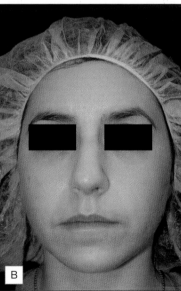

Figure 6.8 Prior to treatment (**A**) and immediately after non-ablative fractional resurfacing (**B**) demonstrating erythema.

The treatments were well tolerated with an average pain score of 4.6 on a scale of 1 to 10.

Given that NAFR was specifically developed to minimize the extent of complications, long-term complications are also extremely rare. Graber and colleagues recently performed the first large-scale study looking at the complications and long-term side effects of NAFR. Consistent with Fisher & Geronemus's study, they also reported a low short-term complication rate. In their study of 422 patients with a total of 961 treatments, the most common complications were acne eruptions (1.87%), HSV outbreaks (1.77%), and erosions (1.35%), all of which occurred with lower frequency than after ablative procedures. Acne outbreaks were more likely to occur in patients who were acne-prone and thus oral antibiotic prophylaxis may be considered in some patients. Other uncommon complications included prolonged erythema and edema.

When similar treatment parameters were used across different skin phototypes, complications were more likely to occur in those that were more darkly pigmented, especially with regards to postinflammatory hyperpigmentation. While an uncommon complication (0.73%), postinflammatory hyperpigmentation (PIH) lasted an average of 51 days, significantly longer than any other complication. Recent studies have shown that, with proper titration of settings, darker-pigmented patients can be treated more safely. While both energy and MTX density determine treatment level, Chan et al provided the first evidence that density of MTZs may specifically increase the risk for PIH. By reducing the density and lengthening the treatment interval, the risk of PIH in darker-skinned patients can be significantly reduced. Sunscreen and hydroquinone use should be implemented both before and after treatment to minimize this risk even further.

While complications, especially long-term ones, are extremely rare, patients should be educated to expect typical side effects including post-treatment erythema, edema, dry skin, and desquamation (Box 6.4).

Advances in technology

The field of fractional resurfacing is relatively new with advances in treatment parameters and new applications for the technology evolving seemingly every month. Since the first fractional resurfacing device was used in 2004, laser systems have continued to be refined and updated. The Fraxel re:store (Solta Medical, Hayward, CA), for example, provides deeper penetration, greater percentage of skin covered, and a variable spot size over the original SR750 model. Non-ablative laser wavelengths have also been broadened significantly with systems utilizing infrared (LuxIR fractional, Palomar Medical Technologies Inc.,

Burlington, MA), and now even radiofrequency. The eMatrix system (Syneron, Irvine, CA), a fractionated bipolar radiofrequency device, utilizes a new concept of sublative rejuvenation. The technology is purported to cause limited epidermal disruption while creating a wider, conical injury zone within the dermis. Although few clinical studies have been done with this newer technology, it is clear that technological advances in fractional photothermolysis will continue to be made as the field evolves even further.

Over-the-counter devices – the future?

Given the tremendous success of in-office devices, several companies are in the process of developing their over-the-counter non-ablative fractional counterparts that are designed for photorejuvenation. PaloVia Skin Renewing Laser (Palomar Medical Technologies, Burlington, MA) was the first handheld, fractional, non-ablative diode laser (1410 nm, 15 mJ, 10 ms pulse duration) to be FDA cleared for the reduction of fine lines and wrinkles around the eyes. With a demonstrated depth penetration of approximately 250 μm, this device has been shown in two pivotal studies to improve facial wrinkle score by at least one grade among 90% of patients after 4 weeks of daily use. On self-assessment in the pivotal phase study, 87% of patients felt they had reduction in the degree of their wrinkles.

Another home-based photorejuvenation device, RéAura (a collaborative effort between Solta Medical, Hayward, CA and Philips, Einthoven, Holland) is currently undergoing further studies and at the time of writing was pending approval by the FDA. This home version of the original Fraxel re:store (Solta Medical, Hayward, CA) is a 1435 nm laser that uses a high-speed scanner and produces fractionated microscopic skin injury at approximately 200 μm. A study of 80 patients who received twice-weekly treatments to face, neck, chest, and arms for 8–12 weeks revealed statistically significant improvement in overall appearance, fine lines, pigmentation, age/sun spots, texture, firmness, and radiance at 1 and 4 weeks after completion of the course of treatment.

Despite the advances made in home fractionated technologies, home devices simply cannot and will not replace office-based non-ablative fractionated devices. Although modest improvement in wrinkles and texture may be observed, the degree of dermal injury cannot match office-based more aggressive devices. Home fractionated devices also carry a significant risk of potential misuse, but the companies that make these devices make every effort to prevent that possibility.

Advanced topics: treatment tips for experienced practitioners

Many patients have both the pigmentary changes and rhytides associated with photoaging. A hybrid approach combining two non-ablative fractional resurfacing wavelengths optimizes outcomes. Alternating 1927 nm with 1550 nm treatments addresses both concerns (Case study 5). An alternative approach uses intense pulsed light (IPL) to address the dyschromia and uneven pigmentation of photoaging while 1550, 1540, or 1440 nm NAFR devices address wrinkling. In a yet unpublished study that we recently performed, the addition of a MaxG IPL (Palomar Medical Technologies, Burlington, MA) treatment immediately prior to the Lux1540 non-ablative resurfacing device yielded significant improvement in photoaging scores when rated by blinded physicians.

CASE STUDY 5
Combination treatment

A 62-year-old female with numerous lentigines and mild rhytides comes in for cosmetic consultation. She has heard that IPL treatment would improve her brown spots. While you agree that IPL would significantly improve her dyspigmentation, you recommended the 1550 nm non-ablative fractionated device alternating with the 1927 nm device instead. Using this treatment strategy, you realize that you can give her a 'bigger bang for her buck' and improve her rhytides as well. She does six treatments (three with each laser) over 6 months and has a very dramatic response. She is extremely pleased with the treatment results.

Conclusion

The science of NAFR has revolutionized our treatment strategies for a host of dermatologic conditions. Coupled with a very favorable side effect profile and minimal downtime, this relatively new technology will continue to gain in popularity. With new devices and modifications to current systems emerging constantly, its applications will also continue to evolve and broaden. Clinical studies demonstrating efficacy and further scientific scrutiny will help continue to advance this technology.

Further reading

Alexiades-Armenakas MR, Dover JS, Arndt KA, 2008 The spectrum of laser skin resurfacing: nonablative, fractional, and ablative laser resurfacing. Journal of the American Academy of Dermatology 58(5):719-737

Bogdan Allemann I, Kaufman J 2010 Fractional photothermolysis – an update. Lasers in Medical Science 25(1):137-144
   This article reviews both ablative and non-ablative fractional photothermolysis. It includes a table of available devices. A little bit cumbersome to read but reviews the literature comprehensively.

Geronemus RG 2006 Fractional photothermolysis: current and future applications. Lasers in Surgery and Medicine 38(3):169-176
   One of the earliest articles discussing the clinical applications of non-ablative fractional photothermolysis through the eyes of one early implementer. Good clinical photos.

Graber EM, Tanzi EL, Alster TS 2008 Side effects and complications of fractional laser photothermolysis: experience with 961 treatments. Dermatologic Surgery 34(3):301-305
   A study with a large population reporting potential complications. The study also documents the safety of non-ablative fractional photothermolysis.

Manstein D, Herron GS, Sink RK, et al 2004 Fractional photothermolysis: a new concept for cutaneous remodeling using microscopic patterns of thermal injury. Lasers in Surgery and Medicine 34:426-438
   The seminal article on the concept of fractional photothermolysis. It includes an excellent background to the technology, mechanism of action, and clinical data.

Marra DE, Yip D, Fincher EF, et al 2006 Systemic toxicity from topically applied lidocaine in conjunction with fractional photothermolysis. Archives of Dermatology 142(8):1024-1026
   A case report of systemic toxicity to topical lidocaine during treatment with non-ablative fractional photothermolysis.

Metelitsa AI, Alster TS 2010 Fractionated laser skin resurfacing treatment complications: a review. Dermatologic Surgery 36(3):299-306
   A good review of treatment of complications with non-ablative fractional photothermolysis.

Narurkar VA 2009 Nonablative fractional laser resurfacing. Dermatologic Clinics 27(4):473-478
   A review of non-ablative fractional photothermolysis and its clinical applications with good before and after photos.

Sherling M, Friedman PM, Adrian R, et al 2010 Consensus recommendations on the use of an erbium-doped 1,550-nm fractionated laser and its applications in dermatologic laser surgery. Dermatologic Surgery 36(4):461-469
   In this article, a group of laser experts provide their recommendations of treatment settings on one particular laser, the Fraxel re:store. An excellent resource to obtain guidelines for treatment settings for new practitioners.

Tierney EP, Kouba DJ, Hanke CW 2009 Review of fractional photothermolysis: treatment indications and efficacy. Dermatologic Surgery 35(10):1445-1461
   A superb review article of both ablative and non-ablative fractional resurfacing with a comprehensive review of the available studies.

7

Laser resurfacing

Jason N. Pozner, Barry E. DiBernardo, Lawrence S. Bass

Summary and Key Features

- Laser resurfacing is a very popular procedure
- A variety of carbon dioxide, Er:YAG and yttrium-scandium-gallium-garnet (YSGG) lasers are included in this category
- Full field means 100% of the treated area is removed to the selected depth
- Fractional means discontinuous portions of the treated area are removed
- Recovery time is linked to amount of damage created
- Fractional treatments have less downtime than full field treatments
- Experience with these lasers is important to outcomes
- Post-treatment care is very important
- Complications can arise with all of these laser treatments

Introduction

Laser resurfacing is a very popular procedure in the United States and worldwide. Data from The American Society of Aesthetic Plastic Surgery collected yearly from core specialists since 1997 through 2010 has shown the rise, fall, and rise again of this procedure as devices have been introduced (Table 7.1). In the mid 1990s carbon dioxide lasers were extremely popular, but toward the turn of the century they fell out of favor and were somewhat replaced by non-ablative technology. Laser resurfacing resurged in the last 5 years with the introduction of fractional lasers.

History

Lasers were introduced into the plastic surgery and dermatology world initially for the treatment of vascular lesions. The introduction of the carbon dioxide laser for skin resurfacing in the mid 1990s rapidly became popular and replaced chemical peels and dermabrasion in many practices. The carbon dioxide laser has a wavelength of 10 600 nm, an absorbing chromophore of water, and is used to vaporize tissue. Continuous mode lasers were initially used, but complications due to excessive depths of ablation and thermal damage led to advances to deliver short laser pulses to the skin to minimize complications. Competing technology delivered either short pulses, each of which contained enough energy to cause tissue ablation (Ultrapulse® laser, Lumenis lasers, Yokneam, Israel) or an optomechanical flashscanner used to scan a continuous laser beam in a spiral pattern (Silk-touch® and Feather-touch® lasers, Lumenis lasers, Yokneam, Israel). Both methods created a tissue exposure time of less than one millisecond, which allowed tissue ablation with limited residual thermal damage of approximately 75–100 µm. Short-term results of eradicating wrinkles and tightening lax tissue were excellent, but longer-term follow-up showed hypopigmentation in a large percentage of patients. These pigmentary complications and the considerable downtime created for the patient led to the demise of 'full field' carbon dioxide laser resurfacing around the turn of the century.

Erbium:YAG lasers (2940 nm) were introduced around 2000 and marketed for superficial resurfacing. Erbium lasers have a higher water absorption coefficient than carbon dioxide lasers (about 10 times more efficient) and ablate tissue with much less thermal damage (5–10 µm). Initial machines were low powered, lacked pattern generators, and needed considerable number of passes and treatment time to achieve deeper depths of ablation. Subsequent systems had more significant power and could be used for efficient deeper resurfacing. There is a linear relationship between the energy delivered and depth of ablation, with approximately 3–4 µm ablated per joule of Er:YAG laser fluence delivered. Complications were fewer, yet downtime appeared to be similar to that of carbon dioxide systems. Conclusions of comparative studies were that the combined depth of ablation and coagulation was the determining factor in length of recovery. Combination systems of carbon dioxide and Er:YAG lasers were popular for a short time (Derma-K®, Lumenis lasers, Yokneam, Israel) with the beams being delivered either sequentially or at the same time.

Variable or long-pulse Er:YAG lasers (Sciton Inc, Palo Alto, CA) allow control over the amount of residual thermal injury produced for a given amount of tissue removal. These variable pulse Er:YAG systems seem to

Table 7.1 Popularity of procedures ASAPS top 10 1997–2010

Year rank	1997	1998	1999	2000	2001	2002	2003	2004	2005	2006	2007	2008	2009	2010
1	Chemical peel	Chemical peel	Chemical peel	Botox	Botox	Botox	Botox	Botox	Botox	Botox	Botox	Botox	Botox	Botox
2	Collagen	Collagen	Botox	Chemical peel	Chemical peel	Microdermabrasion	Laser hair removal	Laser hair removal	Laser hair removal	Hyaluronic acid	Hyaluronic acid	Laser hair removal	Hyaluronic acid	Hyaluronic acid
3	Liposuction	Sclerotherapy	Laser hair removal	Microdermabrasion	Collagen	Collagen	Microdermabrasion	Chemical peel	Hyaluronic acid	Laser hair removal	Laser hair removal	Hyaluronic acid	Laser hair removal	Laser hair removal
4	Blepharoplasty	Lioosuction	Collagen	Collagen	Microdermabrasion	Laser hair removal	Chemical peel	Microdermabrasion	Microdermabrasion	Microdermabrasion	Microdermabrasion	Chemical peel	Microdermabrasion	Laser resurfacing
5	Laser resurfacing	Blepharoplasty	Sclerotherapy	Sclerotherapy	Laser hair removal	Chemical peel	Collagen	Hyaluronic acid	Chemical peel	Laser resurfacing	IPL	Laser resurfacing	Chemical peel	Chemical peel
6	Rhinoplasty	Botox	Liposuction	Laser hair removal	Sclerotherapy	Liposuction	Sclerotherapy	Collagen	Sclerotherapy	Sclerotherapy	Chemical peel	Microdermabrasion	Laser resurfacing	Microdermabrasion
7	Breast augmentation	Rhinoplasty	Microdermabrasion	Liposuction	Liposuction	Sclerotherapy	Liposuction	Laser resurfacing	Laser resurfacing	Chemical peel	Laser resurfacing	IPL	Sclerotherapy	Sclerotherapy
8	Facelift	Breast augmentation	Breast augmentation	Blepharoplasty	Blepharoplasty	Breast augmentation	Breast augmentation	Sclerotherapy	Liposuction	Liposuction	Sclerotherapy	Sclerotherapy	IPL	IPL
9	Botox	Laser resurfacing	Blepharoplasty	Breast augmentation	Breast augmentation	Blepharoplasty	Blepharoplasty	Liposuction	Breast augmentation	Breast augmentation	Liposuction	Breast augmentation	Breast augmentation	Breast augmentation
10	Hair transplantation	Laser hair removal	Laser resurfacing	Rhinoplasty	Rhinoplasty	Rhinoplasty	Rhinoplasty	Breast augmentation	Blepharoplasty	Blepharoplasty	Breast augmentation	Liposuction	Liposuction	Liposuction

produce skin tightening and wrinkle reduction similar to carbon dioxide lasers with a much shorter period of erythema and much lower risk of hypopigmentation. These devices are very popular today.

Other wavelengths for skin resurfacing have been introduced (2780 nm and 2790 nm) (Cutera Lasers, Palomar Lasers) which allow variable degrees of thermal damage and ablation settings but have not had significant commercial success. Plasma skin resurfacing uses nitrogen plasma energy to coagulate a very controlled depth of skin. Healing times and results appear to be similar to Er:YAG lasers. These devices were popular for some time, but were removed from the marketplace due to financial problems of the manufacturer. They were recently reintroduced into the market.

In 2004 Manstein et al introduced the concept of fractional photothermolysis. Full field or traditional laser resurfacing as described above removes the entire skin surface in the area being treated with depth of injury depending upon energy level, whereas fractional laser resurfacing treats a small 'fraction' of the skin at each session, leaving skip areas between each exposed area (Fig. 7.1). This was first performed commercially using non-ablative fluences at 1550 nm (Solta Medical, Mountain View, CA). These non-ablative fractional lasers created a column of thermal damage with intact epidermis. Healing occurred from deeper structures as well as from adjacent structures. This differs from full field resurfacing in which healing occurred from only deeper structures. Deeper treatments (i.e. to the reticular dermis) can safely be performed using this approach than would be tolerated using a full field treatment. Advantages of this approach include avoidance of an open wound and very low risk

of pigment disturbance or scarring. Disadvantages have included the need for multiple treatments and somewhat less clinical response than with full field ablative resurfacing. Since the introduction of the original system there have been many manufacturers that have introduced similar non-ablative fractional devices with wavelengths of 1440 nm, 1540 nm, and 1550 nm. These devices differ in power output, spot size, density, etc. and comparisons of clinical efficacy are difficult, yet similar degrees of tissue injury should produce similar clinical results.

> **Pearl 1**
>
> Full field resurfacing means the entire top layer of the skin (to whatever depth is specified) is removed.

> **Pearl 2**
>
> Fractional resurfacing means a 'fraction' or percentage of the skin is removed (to whatever depth is specified).

Fractional ablative resurfacing with carbon dioxide, erbium, and yttrium-scandium-gallium-garnet (YSGG) systems was introduced with the intent of providing more significant results than non-ablative fractional systems while achieving shorter healing times and complications when compared with full field ablative systems (Fig. 7.2). These devices differ not only in wavelength but in system power, spot size, and amount of thermal damage created adjacent to and deep to the ablated hole. One popular erbium system, the Sciton ProFractional®, allows one to vary the amount of thermal damage similarly to their full field system. Other newer carbon dioxide fractional lasers allow variation of the thermal damage zones (Deka Medical) while others allow superficial and deeper penetration with a single scan (Syneron, Yokneum, Israel). As with the non-ablative fractional systems, direct comparison between devices is difficult as devices differ in power output, spot size, density, and degree of thermal damage, but similar degrees of injury should produce similar clinical results.

The newest wavelength to be introduced into the fractional arena is the Thullium® (1927 nm) by Solta Medical. This non-ablative fractional device is especially effective in removing superficial pigment. Full field ablative resurfacing and both fractional ablative and non-ablative systems remain very popular in clinical use at this time.

Patient selection

Patient selection and a clear understanding of potential complications are important to achieving consistent results. The most common indications for both full field and fractional laser resurfacing are superficial dyschromias, dermatoheliosis, textural anomalies, superficial to deep rhytides, acne scars, and surgical scars. Other conditions that may respond favorably include rhinophyma, sebaceous hyperplasia, xanthelasma, syringomas, actinic

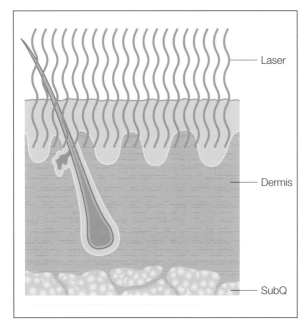

Figure 7.1 Traditional ablative laser resurfacing (full field).

Laser

Dermis

SubQ

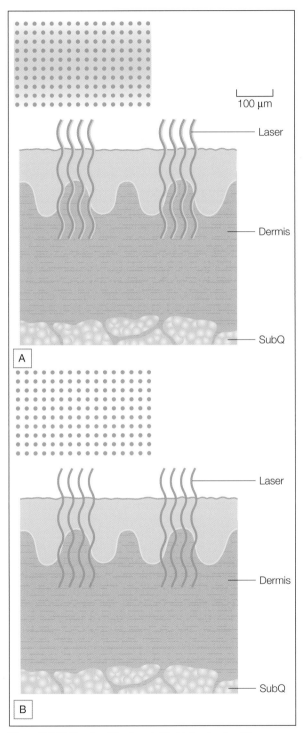

100 μm

Laser

Dermis

SubQ

A

Laser

Dermis

SubQ

B

Figure 7.2 (**A**) Fractional treatment; (**B**) ablative fractional laser treatment.

cheilitis, and diffuse actinic keratoses. Dyschromias such as melasma have been successfully treated with fractional resurfacing but results are not consistent. The usual area for resurfacing is the face, but body and neck skin may be treated with variations of technique. Non-facial areas lack the appendages necessary for skin rejuvenation and treatment must be performed non-aggressively to avoid complications. These devices are generally used with patients with Fitzpatrick skin types I–IV, but can be used in skin types V and VI with modification of technique.

Patient assessment starts at the consultation with observation of the patient's Fitzpatrick skin type, ethnicity, and pathology to be treated. For example, deep acne scarring will not be successfully treated with a single treatment of non-ablative fractional treatment, but mild textural issues may respond to superficial treatment. The next assessment is of the patient's tolerance of healing period 'downtime'. A busy executive with no urgency for end point of clinical results may be able to be treated only with a series of no-downtime non-ablative fractional therapy, whereas the bride's mother looking for maximum improvement in a short time to look her best for her daughter's wedding may need a single session with more aggressive treatment. The last parameter is one not usually discussed in medical journals or book chapters: patient finances. A deep full field resurfacing performed under general anesthesia will be more expensive for the patient then a superficial treatment performed with topical anesthesia. However, in patients with deep rhytides a more aggressive procedure under general anesthesia may be more cost effective than multiple more superficial treatments. Another consideration is laser resurfacing while patients are undergoing other procedures such as facelift, abdominoplasty, or aesthetic breast surgery. These patients often have built-in downtime from other procedures and have the recovery time available for deep resurfacing.

Pearl 3

The patient assessment starts at the consultation with observation of the patient's Fitzpatrick skin type, ethnicity, and pathology to be treated.

Pearl 4

Assessment of patients' ability to subject themselves to 'downtime' of a healing period is important.

Many of us with various devices in our offices can offer patients a plethora of treatment options and this can be very confusing to the patient. An effective consultation will encompass a thorough evaluation of the pathology and provide options to the patients in terms of downtime, efficacy, risks, and cost.

Expected benefits and alternatives

The potential for improvement depends upon the device used and depth and degree of injury produced. There are many options for superficial treatment of texture issues, dyschromias, and superficial rhytides including non-aggressive full field resurfacing with Er:YAG, carbon dioxide, YSGG, or plasma devices or with non-ablative or ablative fractional treatment. Many practitioners are using combination therapy with superficial full field treatment combined with fractional treatment, whereas others are combining fractional ablative and non-ablative therapy and others again are using intense pulsed light therapy combined with resurfacing. Other treatments that may yield similar results for superficial pathologies include light chemical peels such as 15–30% trichloroacetic acid (TCA), intense pulsed light (IPL) devices, and Q-switched lasers (532 nm for dyschromias). We prefer lasers and plasma devices to chemical peels owing to the uniformity and predictability of treatment as the device produces tissue effects with minimal variability from pulse to pulse or patient to patient. The learning curve with lasers is less than with chemical peels due to the predictability of the treatment. Expert chemical peelers may get similar results to laser treatment at a fraction of the laser cost, but years of experience are necessary to achieve consistency of results. Intense pulsed light devices may be used to treat dyschromias and superficial vasculature, but require multiple sessions and do not address textural issues or rhytides. Q-switched lasers (532 nm, 694 nm, and 755 nm) are excellent at removing dyschromias in one session but have resultant erythema that lasts for up to 10 days.

Pearl 5

The potential for improvement depends upon the device used and depth and degree of injury produced.

More significant pathology requires deep treatment to achieve results in a single session. There is still a question of whether repeated superficial therapies with ablative fractional devices will achieve similar results to one more aggressive full field session. Deep ablative full field resurfacing may be performed with either erbium or carbon dioxide systems. YSGG in full field mode and plasma devices do not ablate deep enough to treat more significant pathology. Acne scars appear to respond better to fractional therapy than to full field therapy. Alternative treatments may be deeper chemical peels such as phenol or dermabrasion. The authors feel that lasers provide more consistent and reproducible results than chemical peels or dermabrasion.

Lasers and technical overview

As discussed above, current devices used for ablative laser resurfacing include carbon dioxide, Er:YAG, and YSGG lasers, in both full field and fractional modes, and non-ablative devices in a variety of wavelengths including 1440 nm, 1540 nm, 1550 nm, and 1927 nm (Table 7.2). Some machines offer upgradeable expandable platforms where full field devices and fractional devices are available

Table 7.2 Types of ablative systems

Type of laser	Wavelength		
Full field	10 600 CO_2	2940 erbium	2780 YSGG
Ablative fractional	10 600 CO_2	2940 erbium	2780 YSGG

in one machine whereas other companies offer only isolated full field or fractional devices.

Carbon dioxide full field

Pulsed or scanned full field carbon dioxide lasers were very popular from 1995 to about 2000. These devices were powerful with a typical single pass ablating approximately 75 μm and creating thermal damage of approximately 75–100 μm. This residual area of desiccated tissue reduced the amount of absorbing chromophore (water) and made subsequent passes less efficient, and in fact excessive stacked passes acted as a heat sink and created excessive thermal damage and the potential for scar. Up to three passes were usually performed with the original carbon dioxide resurfacing lasers owing to diminishing efficiency of tissue removal and rapidly increasing risk of complications. The ablated tissue and underlying thermal damage led to long-term collagen changes and tissue remodeling. Healing time with deep full field carbon dioxide laser resurfacing took approximately 10–14 days and caused erythema that typically lasted a few months. Complications of prolonged erythema and delayed hypopigmentation occurred and led to diminished use of these devices. Further complications will be addressed in the complications section.

Er:YAG full field

The erbium:YAG laser (2940 nm) has an absorption coefficient 10 times greater than the carbon dioxide laser and ablates tissue more efficiently and leaves less residual thermal damage (5–10 μm). There is a linear relationship between energy density (fluence) delivered and tissue ablated with 3–4 μm of tissue removed per J/cm^2 and multiple passes can be used to produce deeper tissue removal without additive residual thermal injury. This leads to recovery time of deep full field Er:YAG laser resurfacing of 7 days to full epithelialization followed by 3–6 weeks of erythema. Superficial and deep resurfacing can be performed with these devices with increasing results and increasing recovery times with deeper treatments (Figs 7.3 and 7.4). Complications including hypopigmentation were less than with carbon dioxide laser full field resurfacing.

Variable pulse Er:YAG systems allow a shorter ablative pulse followed by longer subablative pulses to create increasing thermal damage. These devices are typically used to achieve carbon dioxide laser like results, but without the long healing times and complications such as hypopigmentation.

YSGG full field

The 2790 nm yttrium-scandium-gallium-garnet (Pearl®: Cutera, Brisbane, California) provides half the affinity for water as the Er:YAG laser at 2940. This device in full field mode causes ablation of approximately 20–30 μm and residual thermal damage of approximately 20 μm per pass. Healing times and downtime are a few days. Deeper resurfacing is not performed with this device.

Plasma resurfacing

Plasma resurfacing systems create tissue ablation and thermal damage but also a coagulated eschar that remains in place as a biological bandage until underlying skin is reconstituted. Complications and recovery are reported to be less than for aggressive laser skin resurfacing. This device was recently reintroduced to the marketplace (Energist NA Inc., Nyack, NY 10960).

Non-ablative fractional

As previously mentioned, non-ablative fractional resurfacing involves the simultaneous or sequential placement of multiple small spots of laser light onto the surface of the skin with intervening skip areas of unexposed skin. The chromophore used is water and the wavelengths used are 1440, 1470, 1550, and 1540 nm. The lasers create a column of tissue coagulation from 300 to 1200 μm and are called microthermal zones (MTZ). This subject is covered in Chapter 6 and readers are referred there for a more extensive discussion.

Fractional ablative technology

Ablative fractional resurfacing can be performed with carbon dioxide, Er:YAG, and YSGG devices. There are many devices available from many well-known laser manufacturers. Differences in devices are the mode of spot placement – scanning versus stamping, size of holes (width and depth) created, and power output of devices. Differences between fractional carbon dioxide systems, fractional Er:YAG systems, and YSGG systems are similar to their full field counterparts in that the carbon dioxide systems cause leave more residual thermal damage. Newer Er:YAG systems have variable pulse widths, which cause carbon-dioxide-like thermal damage. Re-epithelialization is quicker than with full field ablation and recovery time varies from hours to a few days depending upon depth and density of treatment.

Both ablative fractional and non-ablative fractional devices are used to treat acne and other scars. Multiple

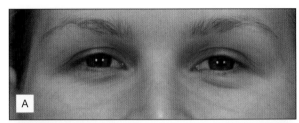
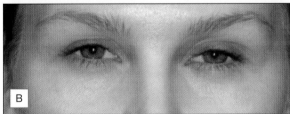

Figure 7.3 Periocular treatment – a 38-year-old female (**A**) before, and (**B**) 3 years after full field variable pulse width Er:YAG laser treatment of the lower lids.

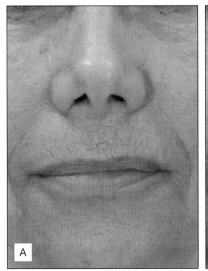
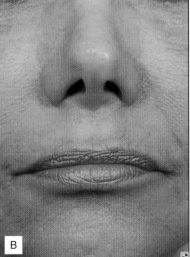

Figure 7.4 Perioral treatment – a 60-year-old woman (**A**) before, and (**B**) 2 years after full field perioral resurfacing with a variable pulse width Er:YAG laser.

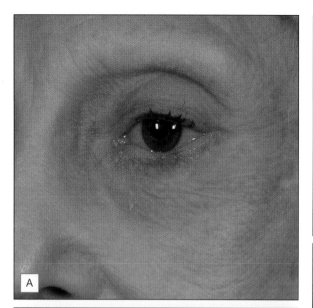

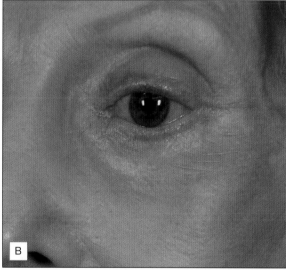

Figure 7.5 A 68-year-old woman with combination fractional Er : YAG resurfacing and fractional 1540 nm non-ablative resurfacing with total coverage of 55%. Time to epithelialization was 4 days. Duration of erythema was 11 days. (**A**) Before, and (**B**) 6 months after treatment.

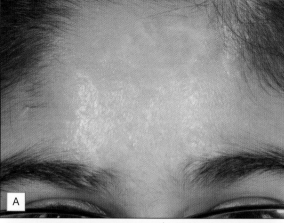

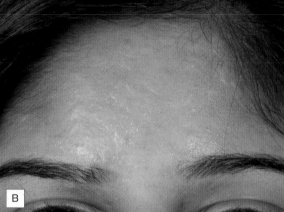

Figure 7.6 (**A**, **B**) This patient had scars of the forehead treated with ablative fractional resurfacing.

treatments are needed and there is no current consensus as to the best technology for this at present. It is very common in our offices to perform combination treatment with superficial full field Er : YAG resurfacing followed by Er : YAG fractional treatment. The superficial Er : YAG treatment improves skin texture and minor irregularities while the fractional treatment is useful for collagen remodeling (Figs 7.5, 7.6).

As fractional CO_2 treatments have been pushed to higher and higher coverages in an attempt to maximize efficacy, healing times predictably have increased. More importantly, complications such as scarring and hypopigmentation have been observed at coverages in excess of 45%. CO_2 resurfacing histology consistently shows a significant component of tissue ablation and coagulation. Efficacious resurfacing is believed to require a significant component of both. One strategy that has been explored to increase coverage percentage and maximize efficacy involves a combination treatment with ablative Er : YAG fractional and non-ablative fractional exposures in a single treatment session. This provides a component of largely ablative exposure with the fractional Er : YAG treatment and a component of coagulation with the non-ablative fractional treatment. Rather than being spatially overlapped as in a fractional CO_2 microthermal zone, the coagulation and ablation are separated. Coverages up to 65% are routinely applied with only a modest increase in healing time and erythema compared with fractional Er : YAG treatment alone and somewhat less than that reported for fractional CO_2. Advantages of this approach include preservation of the short recovery and low incidence of complications seen with fractional Er : YAG treatments and the potential for significant improvement even in perioral rhytides. Disadvantages include the need for two lasers or a single laser platform that offers both options and the time-consuming nature of the treatments (Fig. 7.7).

Overview of treatment strategy

Laser safety

Laser safety is critical to both practitioner and patient. There are excellent published guidelines on laser safety and courses available on the subject. Specifically relevant to ablative and non-ablative resurfacing is the risk of fire and that of eye safety. Fire is an extremely rare occurrence but one must be cognizant not to fire an ablative laser on paper products or gauze. In the operating room, one must be especially careful in the presence of exposed oxygen sources such as nasal cannulas. Some recommend the use of wet towels around the patient's face to prevent a fire hazard.

> **Pearl 6**
>
> Laser safety is critical to both practitioner and patient.

Eye protection is critical for all personnel and the patient. Laser-specific eyewear is used for the treating practitioner and all people in the treatment room. External or internal metal contact lens type eye shields must be used on the patient.

Treatment approach

Patient selection as described above is important to achieve desired results. In summary, patient selection depends upon the following factors:

- skin type
- ethnicity
- pathology – rhytides, acne scars, etc.
- recovery time
- finances
- patient expectations.

> **Pearl 7**
>
> Patient selection as described above is important to achieve desired results. In summary, patient selection depends upon their skin type, ethnicity, pathology (rhytides, acne scars, etc.) tolerance for recovery time, and finances.

There are a few absolute contraindications for laser treatment and some areas of caution.

Absolute contraindications

Active infection

This surgical and elective aesthetic procedure should not be performed in the face of active infection. This is true for bacterial, viral, and fungal infections.

Appendageal abnormality

Laser wounds heal in full field resurfacing from the deep tissues towards the surface from precursor cells in the hair follicles and sebaceous glands, and in fractional resurfacing from those areas and adjacent normal tissue. Patients with abnormalities of the hair follicles and sebaceous glands may have problems with wound healing. Concurrent or recent oral retinoid use is generally considered an absolute contraindication to laser resurfacing. The data is confusing as to whether fractional resurfacing is safe with oral retinoid use. Most experts agree that with return of sebaceous function at 6 months' to 2 years' post-cessation of oral retinoids it is safe to perform deep full field resurfacing. Previously X-ray irradiated skin lacks appendageal structures and as such should not undergo ablative resurfacing procedures.

Extensive electrolysis may also be an absolute contraindication for deep full field resurfacing, but fractional or superficial full field resurfacing should be safe.

> **Pearl 8**
>
> Absolute contraindications for laser resurfacing include infection, appendageal abnormality, deep resurfacing of skin grafts, X-ray-irradiated skin, and extensive electrolysis.

Relative contraindications

Unrealistic expectations are a problem we deal with regularly in plastic surgery and aesthetic dermatology. Laser resurfacing in all its variations can produce some remarkable results but should not be overstated and oversold. Acne scarring especially can be improved dramatically but may require multiple treatments.

Keloid or scarring history

Patients with a history of abnormal scarring may create scars with laser resurfacing. They should be approached with caution and a test treatment area (test spot) may be helpful.

Regional resurfacing in darker-skinned individuals

Deep full field resurfacing in darker-skinned patients may create color differences in adjacent areas. Superficial or fractional regional resurfacing is generally considered safe.

Skin grafts

Care must be taken in patients with skin grafts as the appendages mentioned above are not present in those areas. Resurfacing is routinely used to smooth out the edges; care must be taken with these settings.

Previous deep chemical peel or deep dermabrasion

Caution needs to be taken in patients with previous deep laser or phenol peels or deep dermabrasion as appendages may be damaged and skin may not heal normally.

Figure 7.7 (A–F) Combination treatment with Er:YAG micropeel and Er:YAG fractional. The healing time is 2–3 days; shown are pre-treatment and immediately, day1, day 2, day 3 and 1 week after treatment.

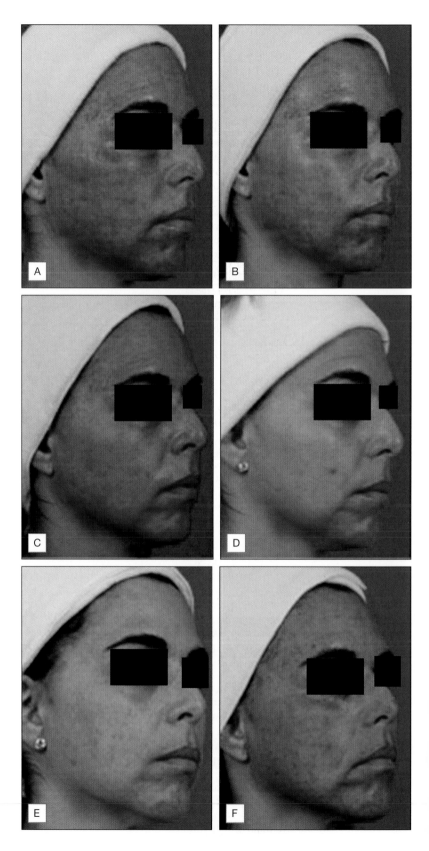

Previous deep laser resurfacing. Caution also needs to be taken in patients who have had deep full field resurfacing as appendages may have been damaged. We routinely resurface patients who have had previous deep carbon dioxide or erbium treatments, but we adjust settings appropriately

History of cold sores/herpes simplex 1

Patients with a strong history of cold sores need a modified prophylaxis regimen compared with patients with no history of cold sores. This should start earlier, by 2–3 days, and extend longer after healing. Even once fully epithelialized, recently resurfaced skin seems to have increased susceptibility to viral infection, unlike bacterial infection risk, which seems largely eliminated by full epithelialization.

> **Pearl 9**
>
> Relative contraindications to laser resurfacing include unrealistic expectations, keloid or abnormal scarring history, regional resurfacing in darker-skinned individuals, and previous deep chemical peel, dermabrasion, or laser resurfacing.

Pre- and post-treatment regimens

Pre-treatment with topical retinoids and bleaching creams is another controversial subject with proponents on either side of this debate with data from chemical peel and laser literature being mixed. Our feeling is that, in full field resurfacing greater than 100 µm in depth, the treated melanocytes are ablated so no benefit to pre-treatment is seen. In superficial full field and fractional resurfacing, pre-treatment may be beneficial in preventing hyperpigmentation. Most recommend cessation of these products a few days prior to treatment.

The use of antiviral prophylaxis is important with ablative resurfacing. There is debate in the literature as to when to start antiviral therapy, with some proposing 3 days prior to treatment whereas others recommend starting on the day of treatment. Most agree that therapy should continue until complete re-epithelialization occurs. This time is laser, patient, and treatment parameter dependent. The use of antiviral therapy with fractional treatments is controversial. We recommend its use as the risk of these medications is low.

Prophylactic antibiotic use is often recommended although we know of no controlled studies of their use. Bacterial infection is extremely rare and is covered in the next section.

After laser treatment there are a myriad of ways to care for the treated skin. For full field procedures, most recommend an occlusive ointment or dressing until epithelialization is complete. We find that occlusive dressings such as Flexzan® work well for carbon dioxide full field resurfacing but are difficult to keep on Er : YAG patients owing to the transudate that occurs following this procedure. Our recommendation is for Aquaphor® or petrolatum until epithelialization is complete then a non-occlusive moisturizer such as Cetaphil® lotion. Deep ablative fractional treatments are usually treated with a similar occlusive regimen for 24–48 hours, although some may prefer a non-occlusive dressing owing to the incomplete epidermal removal.

Use of sunblock is mandatory for all laser-resurfacing patients after epithelialization is complete. We also recommend institution of a skin care regimen after epithelialization is complete and the skin has had a chance to 'calm down'. This may mean a few days for fractional treatments to a few weeks for full field treatments. There are many good skin care regimens appropriate after laser resurfacing. The combination of 4% hydroquinone and low-strength Retin-A® (tretinoin) is still used, although newer regimens with added growth factors are favored by some. The key is to start these regimens slowly to avoid irritation of the skin (see below – dermatitis).

Complications and their treatment

Infection

Infection after laser resurfacing can be viral, bacterial, or fungal. The most well-known complication is due to herpes simplex virus. Many patients have been infected previously and so are carriers. The current recommendation as outlined above is for all patients to be prophylaxed against herpes viral infections. Some patients may avoid taking the anti-viral medications whereas others may experience breakthrough infection (Fig. 7.8). The treatment is early recognition of the infection and treatment with oral antiviral agents. For very severe infections with herpes simplex or zoster intravenous anti-viral medication may be needed.

> **Pearl 10**
>
> Infection after laser resurfacing can be viral, bacterial, or fungal.

Bacterial infection after laser resurfacing using open treatment is uncommon but with increasing methicillin-resistant *Staphylococcus aureus* (MRSA) there have been patients who have had infection after laser resurfacing. The treatment is administration of broad-spectrum antibiotics with culture of the skin and targeted antibiotic treatment after culture results are obtained.

True fungal infection is rare, but infection with yeast (*Candida albicans*) is common (Fig. 7.9). The patient usually presents with an extremely red face with a history of having improvement in the healing and suddenly appearing much redder. Treatment is topical anti-fungal therapy with or without an oral antifungal medication such as fluconazole.

Erythema

Erythema after laser resurfacing is a normal part of the inflammatory healing process. It is directly related to

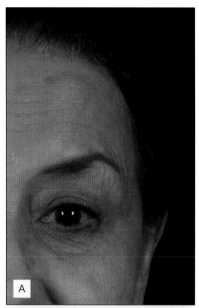

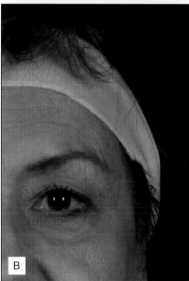

Figure 7.8 A 40-year-old patient who developed candida infection following laser resurfacing.

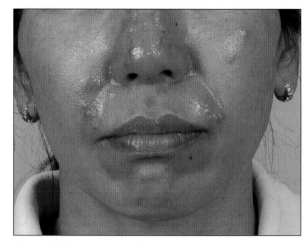

Figure 7.9 Herpes infection following laser resurfacing. Patient failed to take prescribed antiviral medication and noticed these lesions. Patient was treated with valaciclovir 100 mg TID, and responded without scarring.

topical products or to activation of gland function. Acne may be treated with discontinuation of occlusive agents. If this fails, oral antibiotics and/or acne laser treatment with mid-infrared lasers may be used. Milia are treated by nicking the overylying skin with a small-gauge needle and expressing them with a comedo extractor.

Pearl 11

Skin eruptions due to acne or milia are common following laser resurfacing.

Telangiectasia

Increased appearance of telangiectasia after laser resurfacing is common. This is due to eradication of overlying photodamage and unmasking of the vasculature. Treatment is with a vascular laser.

Dermatitis

Two types of dermatitis are seen following laser resurfacing: irritant and allergic. Irritant dermatitis, as mentioned previously, may be due to start of topical skin care treatments such as retinoids too early or too aggressively. Allergic contact dermatitis is due to true allergy, usually to one of the topical agents, but may also be due to one of the oral antibiotics. Treatment for both conditions is discontinuation of the offending agent and application of a mild topical corticosteroid.

Hypopigmentation

This is a dreaded complication of deep laser resurfacing and has been reported both with carbon dioxide and Er:YAG treatments and with full field and fractional

depth of laser resurfacing and to the amount of thermal damage created. Some patients will experience an amount of erythema disproportionate to the treatment. They may be left untreated for the erythema to resolve spontaneously (which it will) or else they may be treated with mild topical corticosteroids, LED treatments, IPL treatments, or with a vascular laser such as a pulsed dye laser.

Skin eruptions

Skin eruptions due to acne or milia are common following laser resurfacing. They may be due to overocclusion with

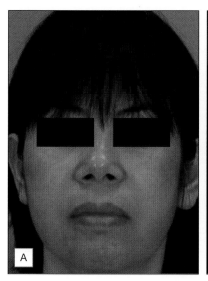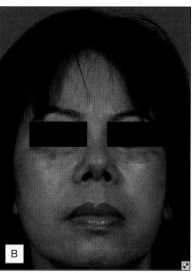

Figure 7.10 A 49-year-old Asian woman who developed hyperpigmentation following Er:YAG resurfacing.

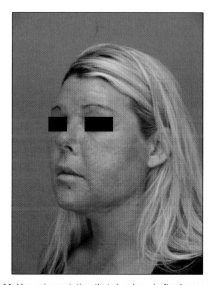

Figure 7.11 Hypopigmentation that developed after laser resurfacing.

treatments. It is not uncommon with deep carbon dioxide resurfacing, with some series reporting up to 70% of patients getting hypopigmentation. It is rare with deep Er:YAG full field resurfacing and very rare with all fractional treatments. There are not many effective treatments, but some have reported improvement with excimer laser therapy. Blending of the noticeable line of demarcation is often helpful (Fig. 7.10).

Hyperpigmentation

Postinflammatory pigmentation (PIH) is a very common problem following laser resurfacing. It is more common in darker skin types and in patients who have had early sun exposure (Fig. 7.11). Prevention as outlined above is key. Treatment is with topical bleaching creams, often combined with retinoids. Failures of this regimen are usually treated with IPL.

> **Pearl 12**
>
> Postinflammatory pigmentation (PIH) is a very common problem following laser resurfacing.

Scarring

Scarring after laser resurfacing may occur owing to overly aggressive full field or fractional treatment, infection, or even scratching by the patient. Full field resurfacing is a controlled first-degree or second-degree burn and anything such as infection may convert that controlled second-degree burn into a third-degree burn with resultant scarring. Overaggressive fractional resurfacing may be due to too deep a treatment, or too much density, creating a full field defect when a fractional treatment was intended. We prefer early treatment of thickened areas that appear to be heading towards scarring with potent topical corticosteroids such as a pulsed regimen with clobetasol. Intralesional corticosteroids, intralesional 5-FU, vascular laser or IPL treatment, and fractional lasers have all been used to improve hypertropic scars after laser resurfacing (Fig. 7.12).

Slow healing

Slow healing has been reported in some cases with re-epithelialization of many months of up to a year. This has led to hypertrophic scarring. This scenario of slow healing may represent an indolent infection. Patients with this scenario should be cultured and potentially biopsied to determine and underlying cause.

Ectropion

Ectropion is caused by laser resurfacing by tightening of the lower eyelid skin in the face of weak lower eyelid

Figure 7.12 A 64-year-old woman who developed a hypertrophic scar after laser resurfacing: (**A**) before, and (**B**) after treatment with intralesional corticosteroids and IPL.

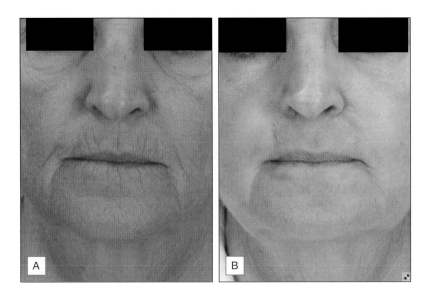

canthal support. A snap test or other measurement of lower eyelid laxity is recommended prior to laser resurfacing. Patients with significant laxity are offered either canthal support surgery (rare) or canthal temporary support (temporary tarsorraphy – common).

Synechia

This is caused by healing of two epidermal surfaces and appears as a line (usually in the lower eyelid). If untreated this may lead to cyst formation. Treatment is to manually stretch the edges of the synechia until the line opens.

Further reading

Bass LS 1998 Erbium:YAG laser skin resurfacing: Preliminary clinical evaluation. Annals of Plastic Surgery 40: 328-334

Bass LS, DelGuzzo M, Doherty S, et al 2009 Combined ablative and non-ablative fractional treatment for facial skin rejuvenation. Lasers in Surgery and Medicine 15(suppl):29

Bogle MA, Arndt KA, Dover JS 2007 Evaluation of plasma skin regeneration technology in low fluence full-facial rejuvenation. Archives of Dermatology 143:168-174

Chan H 2005 Effective and safe use of lasers, light sources, and radiofrequency devices in the clinical management of Asian patients with selected dermatoses. Lasers in Surgery and Medicine 37:179-185

Clementoni MT, Gilardino P, Muti GF, et al 2007 Non-sequential fractional ultrapulsed CO_2 resurfacing of photoaged facial skin: Preliminary clinical report. Journal of Cosmetic and Laser Therapy 9:218-225

Fitzpatrick RE, Rostan EF, Marchell N 2000 Collagen tightening induced by carbon dioxide laser versus erbium:YAG laser. Lasers in Surgery and Medicine 27:395-403

Fisher GH, Geronemus RG 2005 Short-term side effects of fractional photothermolysis. Dermatologic Surgery 31:1245-1249

Friedman PM, Glaich A, Rahman Z, et al 2006 Fractional photothermolysis for the treatment of hypopigmented scars. American Society for Dermatologic Surgery Annual Meeting Presentation, October 2006

Geronemus RG 2006 Fractional photothermolysis: Current and future applications. Lasers in Surgery and Medicine 38:169-176

Kilmer S, Fitzpatrick R, Bernstein E, et al 2005 Long term follow-up on the use of plasma skin regeneration (PSR) in full facial rejuvenation procedures. Lasers in Surgery and Medicine 36:22

Kim KH, Fisher GH, Bernstein LJ, et al 2005 Treatment of acneiform scars with fractional photothermolysis. Lasers in Surgery and Medicine 36:31

Langlois JH, Kalakanis L, Rubenstein AT, et al 2000 Maxims or myths of beauty? A meta-analytic and theoretical review. Psychological Bulletin 126:390-423

Laubach H, Tannous Z, Anderson RR, et al 2005 A histological evaluation of the dermal effects after fractional photothermolysis treatment. Lasers in Surgery and Medicine 26:86

Manstein D, Herron GS, Sink RK, et al 2004 Fractional photothermolysis: a new concept for cutaneous remodeling using microscopic patterns of thermal injury. Lasers in Surgery and Medicine 34:426-438

Morrow PC, McElroy JC, Stamper BG, et al 1990 The effects of physical attractiveness and other demographic characteristics on promotion decisions. Journal of Management 16:723-736

Pozner JN, Goldberg DJ 2006 Superficial erbium:YAG laser resurfacing of photodamaged skin. Journal of Cosmetic Laser Therapy 8(2):89-91

Pozner JN, Goldberg DJ 2000 Histologic effect of a variable pulsed Er:YAG laser. Dermatologic Surgery 26:733-776

Pozner JN, Roberts TL 2000 Variable-pulse width Er:YAG laser resurfacing. Clinics in Plastic Surgery 27:2, 263

Rahman Z, Rokhsar CK, Tse Y, et al 2005 The treatment of photodamage and facial rhytides with fractional photothermolysis. Lasers in Surgery and Medicine 36:32

Rahman Z, Alam M, Dover JS 2006 Fractional laser treatment for pigmentation and texture improvement. Skin Therapy Letters 11:7-11

Tannous ZS, Astner S 2005 Utilizing fractional resurfacing in the treatment of therapy-resistant melasma. Journal of Cosmetic Laser Therapy 7:39-43

Tannous Z, Laubach HJ, Anderson RR, et al 2005 Changes of epidermal pigment distribution after fractional resurfacing: a clinicopathologic correlation. Lasers in Surgery and Medicine 36:32

Tanzi, EL, Alster, TS 2005 Fractional photothermolysis: Treatment of non-facial photodamage with a 1550 nm erbium-doped fiber laser. Lasers in Surgery and Medicine 36:31

Weinstein C, Ramirez OM, Pozner JN 1997 Postoperative care following CO_2 laser resurfacing: Avoiding Pitfalls. Plastic and Reconstructive Surgery 100:1855-1866

Weinstein CW, Ramirez OM, Pozner JN 1997 Carbon dioxide laser resurfacing complications and their prevention. Aesthetic Surgery Journal 17:216-225

Weiss RA, Gold M, Bene N, et al 2006 Prospective clinical evaluation of 1440-nm laser delivered by microarray for the treatment of photoaging and scars. Journal of Drugs in Dermatology 5:740-744

8 Non-surgical body contouring

Andrew A. Nelson, Mathew M. Avram

Summary and Key Features

- Given the epidemic rise of obesity, and the obsession with losing weight and improving our appearance, the treatment of fat and cellulite is a common cosmetic issue
- Fat and cellulite are distinct entities. Cellulite is best considered a hormonally based structural phenomenon of adipocytes and fibrous septae, whereas excess fat is an overabundance of normal adipocytes
- The treatment options for excess fat and cellulite are different and a treatment that improves one may have no discernible impact on the other
- Non-invasive body contouring is a rapidly expanding cosmetic field, with many new technologies recently developed and promising new technologies expected in the near future
- Topical agents, such as retinoids and methylxanthines, have theoretical benefits on the appearance of fat and cellulite, though objective clinical improvements are limited
- Injectable therapies, including mesotherapy and injection lipolysis, are also options for patients
- Physical massage of the affected areas may improve the appearance of fat and cellulite by modulating blood and lymphatic flow. In clinical studies, modest improvements have been observed

- Radiofrequency (RF) devices utilize alternating current to generate ionic flow and localized heat in adipocytes, moderately improving the appearance of fat and cellulite
- High-intensity focused ultrasound (HIFU) can also specifically target adipocytes, thereby improving the appearance and thickness of the fat layer. Recently, a HIFU device was cleared by the FDA for non-invasive waist circumference reduction
- Several laser devices utilizing near-infrared wavelengths, in combination with physical manipulation, have been developed to improve the appearance of fat and cellulite by stimulating dermal collagen formation. Lasers with wavelengths that are selectively absorbed by the adipocytes themselves are currently being developed and studied for potential efficacy
- Cryolipolysis is a novel therapy by which controlled cold exposure (heat extraction) is utilized to selectively damage adipocytes, cause apoptosis, and gradually improve the appearance and thickness of the fat layer over several months following the treatment
- There are few head-to-head studies comparing these different technologies. The ideal treatment option for your patient is best determined by discussing the options with the patient, their ultimate treatment goals, and reaching an informed decision together

Introduction

The treatment of fat is one of the most rapidly expanding areas in medicine and our general culture. Obesity is an unfortunate epidemic in the United States, and weight loss remains a challenging goal for many people. Not only does excess fat present cosmetic challenges to our patients, but it is increasingly obvious that there are also associated significant and dangerous medical effects. In this section, we will focus on non-invasive techniques to improve the appearance of fat and cellulite, the benefits of these technologies, and their limitations. It is important to remember that many of these technologies are relatively new, and

their potential utility will ultimately be determined by well-done randomized scientific studies. Further, none of these devices should be thought of as 'weight loss' devices; rather, modest contouring is typically the most realistic outcome.

Any discussion of treatment of excess fat must begin with liposuction and lasers used in conjunction with liposuction; however, this technique is covered extensively in Hanke & Sattler's Liposuction in this series and will not be reviewed here. Although liposuction remains the true gold standard for treating excess fat, it also requires an invasive procedure with associated discomfort, bruising, and downtime. The last decade has witnessed many new

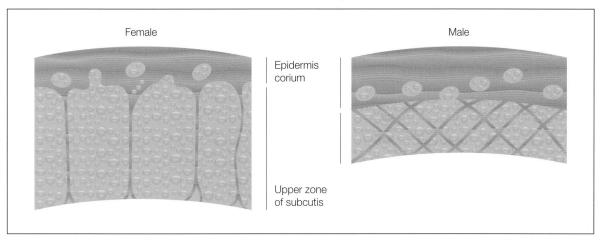

Female   Male

Epidermis
corium

Upper zone
of subcutis

Figure 8.1 Orientation of subcutaneous fibers extending from dermis to fascia in males and females. *Reprinted by permission of Blackwell from Nurnberger F, Muller G 1978 So-called cellulite: An invented disease. Journal of Dermatologic Surgery and Oncology 4:221.*

technologies that have been developed to treat excess adipose tissue through non-invasive techniques. These non-invasive devices utilize a multitude of techniques to improve the appearance of excess adipose tissue, including a reduction in the overall volume of fat, improvement in the appearance of cellulite, and skin tightening.

Fat versus cellulite

Prior to discussing therapeutic options, it is necessary to first differentiate fat and cellulite. Excess fat and obesity are an epidemic, mainly resulting from poor dietary and exercise habits. Fat represents a deposition of excess, but structurally normal, adipose tissue. Cellulite, on the other hand, is best considered a homonally based structural phenomenon of adipose tissue. It is seen almost ubiquitously in post-pubescent females, and rarely in men. As a result of these differences, the techniques and technology that effectively treat excess fat may not have any effect on the appearance of cellulite, and vice versa.

Pearl 1

Excess fat is due to accumulation of normal adipocytes, whereas cellulite is best thought of as a hormonally based structural phenomenon of adipocytes and fat septae. As a result, the evaluation and treatment of these conditions are often divergent.

It is thought that hormones likely play a significant role in the formation of cellulite. Estrogens stimulate lipogenesis and inhibit lipolysis, resulting in adipocyte hypertrophy. Cellulite is typically rare in pre-pubertal females and males of any age, but is extremely common in post-pubertal females. In fact, it has been suggested that cellulite is best considered a secondary sexual characteristic of females. It has also been proposed that cellulite develops in at-risk areas, due to less effective lymphatic and vascular circulation. Exactly how these differences ultimately cause the structural abnormalities of adipose tissue that result in the appearance of cellulite has not been fully elucidated.

Ultrasound and magnetic resonance imaging (MRI) studies have demonstrated the significant structural alterations between male adipose tissue and female cellulite structure. In male adipose tissue, the fibrous septae of the adipose tissue are arranged in an overlapping criss-cross pattern. This theoretically provides greater strength to the overall scaffolding of the adipose tissue and prevents herniation of fat cells. Cellulite, on the other hand, has fibrous septae that are arranged parallel to each other, and perpendicular to the skin surface (Fig. 8.1). This structure is weaker, and allows for the focal herniation of adipose tissue. It is this focal herniation that is thought to cause the classic undulating, lumpy, 'cottage cheese' appearance of cellulite. MRI has demonstrated that women with cellulite do in fact have fibrous septae that are oriented in parallel to each other, although these septae may actually be more similar to pillar-like columns (Figs 8.2 and 8.3). In addition to this structural difference, MRI, ultrasound, and biopsies have also demonstrated that women with cellulite typically have an undulating, lumpy interface between the adipose tissue and the dermis, known as *papillae adiposae* (Fig. 8.4). This interface also likely contributes to the appearance of cellulite.

It is less well established whether excess adipose tissue contributes to the appearance of cellulite. There are many thin females who have the appearance of cellulite on their bodies, whereas some heavier females may display only a subtle appearance of any cellulite. It is likely that excess adipose tissue may predispose or exacerbate the cellulite, but it is less likely that excess adipose tissue alone is a driving factor. We believe that excess fatty tissue and cellulite should be considered as two distinct entities, and that they should be evaluated and treated as such.

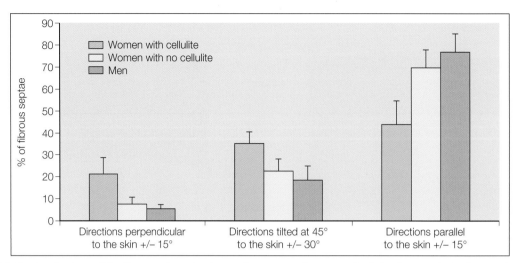

Figure 8.2 Structured patterns of the fibrous septae network according to sex and presence of cellulite. Our quantitative findings give more evidence about the heterogeneity in the directions of the septae, and highly suggest that modeling the 3D architecture of fibrous septae as a perpendicular pattern in women but tilted at 45 degrees in men would be an oversimplification. *Reprinted by permission of Blackwell from Querleux B, Cornillon C, Jolivet O, Bittoun J 2002 Anatomy and physiology of subcutaneous adipose tissue by in vivo magnetic resonance imaging and spectroscopy: relationships with sex and presence of cellulite. Skin Research and Technology 8:118-124.*

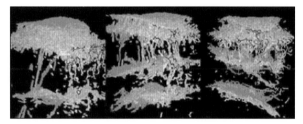

Figure 8.3 Visualization of the 3D architecture of fibrous septae in subcutaneous adipose tissue: (**A**) woman with cellulite, (**B**) normal woman, and (**C**) man. *Reprinted by permission of Blackwell from Querleux B, Cornillon C, Jolivet O, Bittoun J 2002 Anatomy and physiology of subcutaneous adipose tissue by in vivo magnetic resonance imaging and spectroscopy: relationships with sex and presence of cellulite. Skin Research and Technology 8:118-124.*

Evaluation of fatty tissue and cellulite

Body mass index (BMI = person's weight in kilograms divided by the square of their height in meters), remains the classic method for determining obesity. However, this may be an over-simplification, as it does not necessarily take into account the patient's mixture of muscle and adipose tissue or their overall body type. Furthermore, many patients presenting for non-invasive body sculpting may be in very good shape overall with only a few small problem areas such as the thighs or flanks. Although BMI may be a useful tool for defining obesity in large populations, we do not find it particularly useful in our practice. More commonly, we utilize measurements such as thigh circumference, waist circumference, skinfold thickness, visual assessment, and photographic comparisons pre- and post-procedure in our practice, as these more typically reflect the patient's ultimate clinical presentation and outcome.

Pearl 2

BMI is a simple tool to assess overall body habitus. However, BMI is often not the best method to assess localized areas of fat excess and is not often used in our clinical assessments. Furthermore, obese patients (BMI > 30) are often not good candidates for non-invasive body contouring and may require diet, bariatric, or other surgical interventions.

Cellulite can similarly be assessed with various measurements and definitions. Typically, direct observation with side lighting is the simplest and most effective assessment. Based upon these observations, a relatively simple scoring system for the appearance of cellulite has been described (Table 8.1).

More recently, technologies such as ultrasound, MRI, and electrical conductivity have been utilized to assess adipose tissue and cellulite. These technologies are often employed in clinical trials in order to assess the potential efficacy of a novel therapeutic option. However, they are typically not necessary in the evaluation and management of patients' in general practice.

Therapeutic options

There are many different technologies and techniques for non-invasive body sculpting. Options include: topical creams, injectable agents, physical manipulation, lasers and light sources, and cryolipolysis. The best option for your patient is dependent on their clinical presentation, treatment goal, and most importantly, their preferences. It is important to emphasize that none of these treatments provides more than a modest, local contouring benefit in most instances.

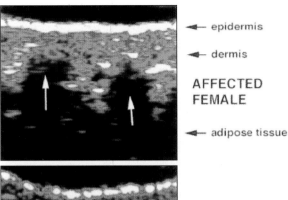

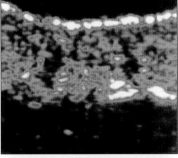

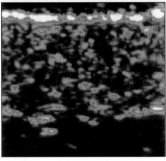

← epidermis

← dermis

AFFECTED FEMALE

← adipose tissue

UNAFFECTED FEMALE

UNAFFECTED MALE

Figure 8.4 Color sonographs of the thigh of an affected woman, an unaffected woman, and an unaffected man. Note the extrusion of adipose tissue into the dermis of the affected individual. *Reprinted by permission of Pierard-Franchiemont C, Pierand GE, Henry F, et al 2000 A randomized, placebo controlled trial of topical retinal in the treatment of cellulite. American Journal of Clinical Dermatology 1:369–374.*

Table 8.1 Cellulite classification

Grade I	No or minimal skin irregularity upon standing, pinch test, or muscle contraction
Grade II	No or minimal skin irregularity upon standing. Dimpling becomes apparent by pinching or muscle contraction
Grade III	Classic skin dimpling at rest with palpable, small subcutaneous nodularities
Grade IV	More severe puckering and nodularity

Topical creams

A simple trip to any cosmetic aisle or beauty store demonstrates that there are numerous topical creams that purport to melt away fat and cellulite. Generally speaking, the active ingredients in these products are thought to stimulate improved circulation, improve lymphatic drainage, or cause lipolysis to improve the appearance of fat and cellulite. Unfortunately, many of these agents have little or no evidence to support their claims.

Pearl 3

Many topical creams are advertised to improve the appearance of fat and cellulite. These claims, in our view, should be regarded skeptically.

Topical retinol compounds have long been a mainstay in cosmetic regimens owing to their ability to stimulate neocollagenosis. Topical retinoids could theoretically improve the appearance of cellulite by increasing collagen deposition and promoting glycosaminoglycan synthesis, thereby resulting in stronger and denser fibrous septae. In clinical studies, the results have been modest. Kligman et al conducted a double-blind study of 20 patients who applied topical retinol twice daily for 6 months, and demonstrated a clinical improvement. A further study of 15 patients by Pierard-Franchimont et al demonstrated a phenotypic shift of connective tissue cells, but no visible improvement in overt cellulite appearance following 6 months of application of topical retinol. Thus, although topical retinoids may be of benefit in improving the appearance of fat and cellulite, this benefit is likely modest at best.

Methylxanthines, such as aminophylline, have also been reported to be effective in treating cellulite. These agents act as phosphodiesterase inhibitors, which, when applied, result in an increase in cyclic adenosine monophosphate (cAMP) levels. This increase in cAMP could theoretically activate hormone-sensitive lipase and thereby stimulate lipolysis in the treated areas. Although there were some initial promising results, other studies have failed to document substantial clinical improvements in the appearance of fat and cellulite.

Numerous herbal therapies have also been reported to be effective in treating fat and cellulite (Table 8.2). Many of these herbal supplements have not undergone rigorous testing to determine their efficacy, and their clinical utility remains to be fully elucidated.

Injectable agents

Many different agents have been injected with the goal of dissolving excess adipose tissue and cellulite. Mesotherapy, or intradermotherapy, is performed by the direct injection of pharmacologic agents into the dermal–subcutaneous junction of the skin. This procedure is purported to work by acting directly on the adipocyte to

Table 8.2 Herbal treatments for cellulite

Herbal name	Concentration (%)	Parts of the plant	Main constituents	Mechanism of action
Bladderwrack	1	Whole dried thallus		Stimulates vascular flow
Butcher's broom	1–3	Rhizome and flowering tops	Saponins, ruscogenin and neororuscogenin	Improves microcirculation
Ginkgo biloba	1–3			Improves microcirculation
Cynara scolymus or artichoke		Leaves, flower heads and roots	Enzymes, cynarin, ascorbic acid, caffeoylquinine acid derivatives, and flavonoids	Reduces edema and promotes diuresis
Common ivy	2	Dried leaves, stems	Saponins (especially hederin)	Improves venous and lymphatic drainage, and reduces edema
Ground ivy	2		Flavonoids, triterpenoids, and phenolic acids	Increases microvascular flow
Indian or horse chestnut	1–3	Seeds, shells	Triterpenoid saponins and flavones, coumarins and tannins	Reduces lysosomic enzyme activity and capillary permeability
Sweet clover	2–5	Flowers and leaves	Coumarin	Reduces lymphatic edema and capillary permeability
Centella asiatica	2–5	Leaves and roots	Asiaticoside, madecassic acid, asiatic acid	Anti-inflammatory and potent healing effects
Red grapes	2–7		Tannins, procyanidins	Contains antioxidants that decrease lipid peroxidation and increase permeability of lymphatic and microarterial vessels
Corynanth yohimbe, *Pausinystalia youhimbe*, and *Rauwolfia serpentine*		Leaves, shells, roots	Yohimbe	Stimulates metabolism of fat cells
Papaya	2–5	Fruits, leaves	Papain and bromelain (proteolytic enzymes)	Anti-inflammatory effects, decreases edema

promote lipolysis or adipolysis, and thereby improve the appearance of fat and cellulite. Closely related, but separate, is a technique known as injectable lipolysis, in which detergents like bile salts (i.e. sodium deoxycholate) are injected into the subcutis to chemically ablate adipose tissue. Although some of these injectibles are currently being developed, none is currently cleared by the FDA and a full discussion of these emerging techniques and agents is beyond the scope of this chapter.

Physical manipulation

Endermologie® (LPG Systems, Valence, France) is an FDA-cleared device that massages and kneads the skin to improve the appearance of cellulite. The device utilizes two rollers, as well as positive and negative pressure, to manipulate the patient's skin. The technique is thought to stimulate blood and lymphatic flow, thereby altering the architecture of the fat and improving the appearance of

cellulite. In clinical studies, modest clinical improvements have been observed. A study by Gulec, of 33 women who were treated with Endermologie® for 15 sessions, demonstrated a statistically significant improvement in the appearance of cellulite as assessed by a visual scale; however, few of the patients (5 of the 33) actually demonstrated clinical improvement. A study by Collis et al compared twice weekly treatment with Endermologie® to a combination treatment of aminophylline cream and Endermologie®. The authors concluded that Endermologie® is not an effective treatment of cellulite, although 10 out of 35 patients with Endermologie®-treated legs reported that their cellulite appearance improved. In summary, Endermologie® may result in modest improvements in the appearance of fat and cellulite in some patients, though it likely requires continuing treatments to maintain any improvement. Home therapy units, such as Well Box®, are available to facilitate ongoing convenient treatment, and may be of benefit to patients.

Pearl 4

Physical manipulation, such as Endermologie®, may result in modest temporary improvement in the appearance of cellulite, but the results are transient and often require ongoing treatments. At-home units may be a convenient and effective option for patients.

Subcision is a relatively simple technique to attempt to improve the appearance of cellulite. A special notched catheter needle is placed into the subcutis of the affected area. The catheter is then physically manipulated by pushing and pulling, in order to break up the fibrous stranding and tethers that are thought to be responsible for the appearance of cellulite. By destroying these fascial tethers, the appearance of cellulite is thought to improve. Side effects such as ecchymosis and edema are common. The clinical utility of this method likely varies depending on the skill of the surgeon, and its clinical utility remains to be fully determined.

Liposuction remains the gold standard treatment for physical removal of excess adipose tissue. A full discussion of liposuction techniques is beyond the scope of this discussion. It is important to note, however, that liposuction's role in the treatment of cellulite is not well established. There are reports of liposuction improving, as well as worsening, the appearance of cellulite. Given the architectural component of cellulite physiology, it is not unexpected that bulk fat removal alone would not improve its appearance.

Pearl 5

Liposuction is the gold standard for large volume fat removal, but is much less reliable for small, localized fat excess. Liposuction is best in patients with >1 inch (25 mm) of pinched skin and fat on exam. Liposuction is also less reliable for the treatment of cellulite.

CASE STUDY 1

A female patient presents to discuss non-invasive fat treatment options. She is 35 years old, weighs 185 pounds (84 kg) and is 5′4″ (1.63 m) tall. She has also developed early onset type II diabetes. She has previously tried to lose weight with diet and exercise, but has been previously unsuccessful. She was recently evaluated by her PCP, who encouraged her to lose weight to improve her diabetes and overall health. She presents to your office, as she would like a procedure to treat her excess adipose tissue.

This patient has a common misconception that non-invasive fat treatment can substitute for large-scale weight loss. This patient's BMI is 31.8, which defines her as obese. Furthermore, she already has a medical comorbidity, diabetes, associated with her obesity. This patient absolutely needs help losing weight and improving her medical health, particularly since she has tried and failed previous weight loss strategies.

She should be referred to a bariatric weight loss program in order to help her achieve her goals of weight loss.

If she is interested in a procedure to help improve her chances of successfully losing weight, this patient may be a good candidate for laparoscopic banding, partial gastrectomy, or gastric bypass. Once the patient has lost weight and is closer to her ideal weight, if she continues to have focal trouble spots of excess fat, she may benefit from a non-invasive body sculpting procedure at that time.

Radiofrequency devices

Radiofrequency (RF) devices pass sinusoidal, alternating current (AC) through tissue to generate heat. The AC causes ionic flow in the treatment tissue, thereby creating heat from molecular friction. In essence, the tissue itself is the source of the heat, rather than the actual device. As a result, RF is thought to cause localized heating of a targeted tissue mass, while limiting the potential for collateral spread of energy, neuromuscular reaction, or electrolysis. Adipose tissue has high tissue resistance and a relatively low heat transfer coefficient; as a result, adipose tissue can be readily heated and the heat will be predominantly confined to the adipocytes. Recently, many RF devices have been advertised to improve the appearance of fat and cellulite.

The VelaSmooth® and VelaShape® (Syneron Medical Ltd, Irvine, CA) devices combine physical manipulation (massage and suction), with bipolar RF energy and infrared light (700–2000 nm) to treat excess fat and cellulite. It has been proposed that these devices improve fat and cellulite by heating the subcutaneous tissue and fat, thereby causing increased localized blood flow and lipolysis. In a randomized clinical study by Nootheti et al, comparing the VelaSmooth® device with another laser device for cellulite (TriActive®, Cynosure Inc., Westford, MA), patients were treated twice weekly for 6 weeks. Following the treatments, patients were observed to have an improvement in the upper and lower thigh circumference, as well as in the appearance of cellulite (Figs 8.5 and 8.6). Seventy-five percent of patients were observed to have an improvement, when comparing pre- and post-treatment photographs, but the results were modest. There were no statistically significant differences in the efficacies of the two devices. Bruising can occur following treatment with the VelaSmooth® device, and was more common with this device than the Triactive® device (Fig. 8.7).

Pearl 6

Bruising is a common side effect of laser and light source treatments for fat. Most commonly, the bruising is related to the vacuum pressure and physical manipulation of the device, rather than the actual laser.

Unipolar, volumetric RF devices with more diffuse, deep heating have also been advocated for the treatment of fat and cellulite. Goldberg et al treated 30 patients

Figure 8.5 A 47-year-old woman (**A**) before, and (**B**) after six treatments with the VelaShape® device. *Photos courtesy of Neil S. Sadick, MD. Reprinted with permission from Sadick NS 2010 VelaSmooth and VelaShape. In Goldman MP, Hexsel D (eds) Cellulite: pathophysiology and treatment, 2nd edn. Informa Healthcare, New York, NY, p 108-114.*

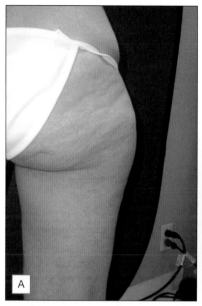
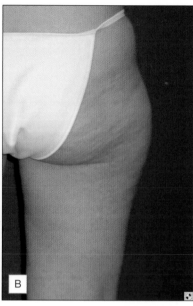

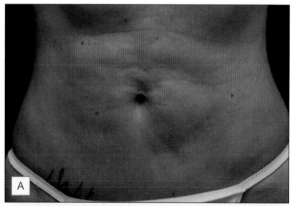
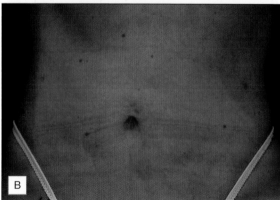

Figure 8.6 A 37-year-old woman (**A**) before, and (**B**) after seven treatments with the VelaShape® device. *Photographs courtesy of Neil S. Sadick, MD. Reprinted with permission from Sadick NS 2010 VelaSmooth and VelaShape. In Goldman MP, Hexsel D (eds) Cellulite: Pathophysiology and Treatment, 2nd edn. Informa Healthcare, New York, NY, p 108-114.*

with a unipolar RF device (Accent®, Alma Lasers US, Buffalo Grove, IL) every other week for a total of six treatment sessions. A decrease in mean leg circumference of 2.45 cm was observed, although the study was limited due to a lack of comparative controls. In general, circumference is not a good end point to assess cellulite improvement. Histological specimens did demonstrate dermal fibrosis that could explain the clinical improvement, although the results were limited. Further clinical studies are necessary to establish the potential role for these RF devices.

Ultrasound devices

Patients are typically accustomed to the diagnostic utility of ultrasound imaging devices. More recently, focused ultrasound devices have been developed to treat the subcutis and adipocytes. These devices have shown promising initial results, and long-term clinical studies are ongoing. Recently, the Liposonix® device (Solta Medical Inc., Hayward, CA) was FDA cleared for non-invasive waist circumference reduction. Additional ultrasound devices are currently being evaluated for possible FDA clearance.

A study by Jewell et al of the Liposonix® device (Solta Medical Inc., Hayward, CA) documented significant improvement following a single treatment session. One hundred and eighty patients were randomized to either a sham treatment or one of two doses of high intensity focused ultrasound. Twelve weeks after the ultrasound treatment, the patients treated with the higher dose had achieved a statistically significant improvement in waist circumference compared with the sham group (−2.44 cm versus −1.43 cm). Patients were observed to have 'improved' or 'much improved' outcomes as assessed by

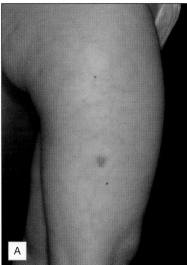

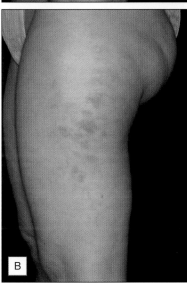

Figure 8.7 Purpura after treatment with (**A**) Triactive® and (**B**) Velasmooth®. *Reproduced with permission from: Nootheti PK, Magpantay A, Yosowitz G, Calderon S, Goldman MP 2006 A single center, randomized, comparative, prospective clinical study to determine the efficacy of the Velasmooth system versus the Triactive system for the treatment of cellulite. Lasers in Surgery and Medicine 38:908-912.*

of 164 patients was conducted by Teitelbaum et al to determine the efficacy of the device; 137 patients underwent one ultrasound treatment to the abdomen, thighs, or flanks; 12 weeks later, mean circumference reductions of 2.3 cm (abdomen), 1.8 cm (thighs), and 1.6 cm (flanks) were observed. The majority (77%) of the improvement in circumference was noted to occur within the first 14 days following the treatment.

Ultrasound technologies represent a new and evolving area within the field of non-invasive fat treatment. Initially, many of the ultrasound technologies were incorporated into liposuction treatments, known as ultrasound-assisted liposuction (UAL). However, more recently, high-intensity focused ultrasound is being developed as a stand-alone non-invasive treatment for improving the appearance of fat and cellulite. These devices require further clinical study in order to determine their long-term efficacy and safety profile. Nevertheless, they represent an exciting and promising opportunity within this field.

Lasers and light sources

Many different light sources and lasers have been advocated as therapeutic options for fat and cellulite. Many are incorporated into liposuction procedures, known as laser-assisted liposuction (LAL); these devices, however, still require invasive liposuction. Other devices have been marketed as being effective, non-invasive therapies for fat and cellulite, though definitive objective evidence of their efficacy may be lacking. Several devices that are advertised to improve fat and cellulite do not actually affect the adipocytes themselves, but rather target the dermis in an attempt to stimulate collagen formation/remodeling. Devices with wavelengths in the near-infrared region, as well as intense pulsed light (IPL) sources, fall into this category.

The TriActive® device (Cynosure Inc., Bedford, MA) combines deep tissue massage and suction (similar to Endermologie®), with contact cooling and a low-intensity diode laser (808 nm). The device purports to increase lymphatic drainage, improve blood flow, and simultaneously tighten skin in the treated areas, which is thought to improve the appearance of cellulite. Patients typically are treated with the device twice weekly, with a progressive improvement following the treatments. In clinical studies, patients were noted to achieve improvement in the appearance of cellulite, as well as objective improvement in hip and thigh circumferences. Subjective improvement included reduction in the appearance of skin dimpling, improvement in the overall contour of the limb, and improvement in overall skin texture (Fig. 8.8). The treatments were well tolerated, although many patients (~20%) developed mild bruising.

The SmoothShapes® device (Eleme Medical, Merrimack, NH) combines two different wavelengths with a massage system similar to Endermologie®. The 915 nm diode wavelength is reported to cause liquefaction of the fat, while the 650 nm wavelength is thought to improve

physicians, and patients were satisfied with their treatments. The procedure is often painful, and bruising and edema develop after treatments. However, no significant laboratory abnormalities were observed following treatment, including: lipid profiles, markers of inflammation, coagulation, liver or renal function, hematologic assessments, or blood chemistry.

The Ultrashape Contour I® (Ultrashape Ltd, Tel Aviv, Israel) is being used in Europe and the United Kingdom for the treatment of excess adipose tissue. At the time of writing, the Ultrashape I® Contour device was not FDA cleared. A prospective, non-randomized, controlled trial

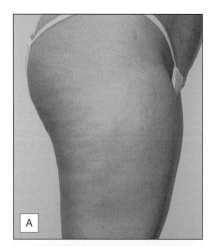

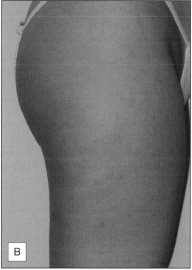

Figure 8.8 Cellulite treatment with Triactive®: subject (**A**) before, and (**B**) following 10 treatments. *Reproduced with permission from: Boyce S, Pabby A, Chuchaltkaren P, Brazzini B, Goldman MP 2005 Clinical evaluation of a device for the treatment of cellulite: Triactive. American Journal of Cosmetic Surgery 22:233-237.*

fat membrane permeability, thereby allowing the adipocytes to be mobilized to the interstitium. Multiple passes with the device are typically performed during a treatment session, with 2–3 sessions being performed each week for best results. In clinical studies by Lach & Kulick, the SmoothShapes® device resulted in reduction of the thickness of the subcutaneous fat pad, as assessed by MRI. The device was well tolerated with no significant associated adverse events.

The VelaSmooth® and VelaShape® (Syneron Medical Ltd, Irvine, CA) devices, as discussed previously, combine physical manipulation with radiofrequency energy, as well as infrared energy, to facilitate a multimodality approach to fat and cellulite treatment. The efficacy of these devices was previously discussed in the above section on radiofrequency. In the future, more devices may approach fat and

cellulite treatment through this multimodality approach in an effort to achieve greater efficacy.

Fat-specific lasers are also being studied, which would selectively target adipocytes themselves rather than modulating the fascia or dermis. Wavelengths such as 1210 nm and 1720 nm are intriguing, given the relative absorption peaks of lipids in these regions. At the present time, however, no commercial laser device that selectively targets fat via selective photothermolysis has been FDA approved.

Cryolipolysis

CoolSculpting® (Zeltiq Aesthetics, Pleasanton, CA) is a relatively novel FDA-cleared device for non-invasive fat reduction; it utilizes cryolipolysis technology to selectively cool fat, extracting energy, and ultimately causing apoptosis. The treatment consists of applying a treatment applicator to the patient's desired treatment area, typically the flank 'love handle', the back 'back fat pads' or the abdomen 'muffin top'. A moderate vacuum is then created by the device, drawing the tissue between the treatment plates and clamping down on local cutaneous blood flow to increase the efficiency of cooling. The treatment cycle lasts up to 60 minutes per cycle, at the conclusion of which the skin appears cool, firm, and erythematous. The tissue is typically molded into the shape of the treatment applicator. At the conclusion of the treatment, the physician massages the area gently to break up any crystallized adipocytes. Over the next several weeks to months, the adipocytes are mobilized and eliminated by the body.

CASE STUDY 2

A 53-year-old female, who is 5'6" (1.68 m) tall and weighs 145 pounds (66 kg), presents for treatment of small pockets of excess fat around her abdomen. She would like to discuss non-invasive treatment options, as she is concerned about the risks of invasive surgery.

This patient's BMI is 23.4, which is within the normal range. She does have localized pockets of excess adipose tissue below the umbilicus, without substantial skin redundancy. This patient could be a good candidate for localized, tumescent liposuction, if she desired. However, she states she does not want an invasive procedure. After discussing options, she elects to have the area treated with CoolSculpting®. The proposed treatment area is marked (a separate, but representative patient is shown in **Fig. 8.9A**). Due to the size, two applications in the same treatment session will be necessary to treat the complete area, each marked with an X (**Fig. 8.9B**). A pinch test is performed to insure that the area can be effectively elevated in the device (**Fig. 8.9C**). The patient undergoes treatment with no adverse effects.

It is important to remind the patient that the full effect of the treatment will not be visible for 2–3 months. In the post-procedure photo, taken 16 weeks after the patient's single cryolipolysis treatment session, a noticeable reduction in the volume and appearance of the abdominal fat 'muffin top' is clearly observable (**Fig. 8.9D, E**).

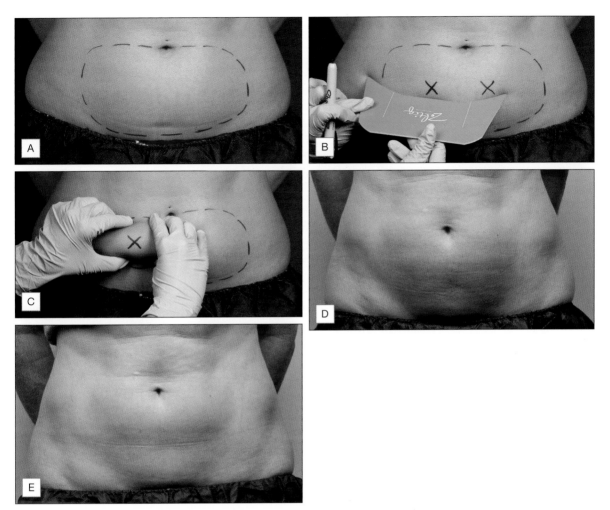

Figure 8.9 A female patient presents for treatment of a localized accumulation of excess adipose tissue below the umbilicus. (**A**) The treatment area is outlined by the treating physician. (**B**) The treating physician then compares the size of the treatment applicator with the planned treatment area. In this case, given the size of the planned treatment area, two treatment applications will be necessary to treat the entire area. The center of each treatment area is marked with an X. (**C**) A pinch test is performed on the area prior to the treatment to insure that the area can be effectively elevated in the device. (**D**) A baseline photograph of the treatment area is taken prior to the patient's cryolipolysis treatment. (**E**) The patient is shown 16 weeks after a single cryolipolysis treatment to the abdomen. Note the significant improvement in the appearance of the thickness of the fat pad. *Photos (**A–C**) courtesy of Zeltiq Inc., Pleasanton, CA. Photos (**D**) and (**E**) courtesy of Dr Flor Mayoral, Coral Gables, FL and Zeltiq Inc., Pleasanton, CA, USA.*

In a recent clinical study, a significant reduction in the thickness of the fat in the treatment area was observed following a single CoolSculpting® treatment (mean fat pad thickness reduction of 22.4%, as measured on high-resolution ultrasound). Of the 32 patients in the study, all had achieved a significant visible contour improvement following a single treatment. The best results were in patients with localized, discrete fat bulges. Another study demonstrated that 79% of patients reported clinical improvement in the appearance of their abdominal fat 2–4 months following a single CoolSculpting® treatment. In these studies, the treatment was well tolerated. Patients may bruise following the procedure, likely due to the vacuum effect of the device. Many patients develop transient altered sensation, numbness or even sharp pain in the treatment area, lasting up to 2 weeks. In rare instances, the pain is sufficient to warrant treatment with pain medications. No significant changes in lipid profiles or liver function tests following cryolipolysis have been demonstrated in either the initial animal studies or human clinical studies. There is a cost for each treatment cycle for the treating physician (i.e. disposable). Finally, no cases of scarring or ulceration of the skin have been reported to date.

Pearl 7

Following a CoolSculpting® treatment, gentle massage of the treated area should be performed to break up crystallized adipocytes and improve the efficacy of the treatment.

Cryolipolysis represents a novel, non-invasive treatment option for fat. Patients can undergo a safe, effective, and simple procedure, which will gradually reduce the appearance of unwanted fat over the following 2–4 months. It should be noted that the device works best for localized, discrete fat bulges and is not intended for the treatment of obesity or as a substitute for large-volume liposuction.

Conclusion

The field of non-invasive body contouring has evolved rapidly in the last several years. Although liposuction and surgical procedures remain the gold standard for patients seeking large-volume fat removal, these non-invasive options represent simple procedures with limited or no downtime to improve the appearance of fat and cellulite. Topical creams, injectable agents, and physical manipulation all represent options for patients seeking non-invasive treatments.

Within the realm of lasers and light sources, there are numerous options for patients including radiofrequency, focused ultrasound, lasers, and cryolipolysis. These technologies are relatively new, and the ultimate treatment efficacy will continue to be established through controlled clinical trials. At the present time, head-to-head studies comparing the devices are limited and, as a result, it is difficult to definitively compare the efficacy of the devices. The best option for your patient ultimately depends on their treatment goals and expectations.

Further reading

Avram MM 2004 Cellulite: a review of its physiology and treatment. Journal of Cosmetic and Laser Therapy 6:181-185

Collis N, Elliot LA, Sharpe C, et al 1999 Cellulite treatment: a myth or reality: a prospective randomized, controlled trial of two therapies, endermologie and aminophylline cream. Plastic and Reconstructive Surgery 104(4):1110-1114

Dover J, Burns J, Coleman S, et al 2009 A prospective clinical study of noninvasive cryolypolysis for subcutaneous fat layer reduction – Interim report of available subject data. Presented at the Annual Meeting of the American Society for Laser Medicine and Surgery, April 2009, National Harbor, MD

Goldberg DJ, Fazeli A, Berlin AL 2008 Clinical, laboratory and MRI analysis of cellulite treatment with a unipolar radiofrequency device. Dermatologic Surgery 34(2):204-209

Güleç AT 2009 Treatment of cellulite with LPG endermologie. International Journal of Dermatology 48:265-270

Hamilton EC, Greenway FL, Bray GA 1993 Regional fat loss from the thigh in women using 2% aminophylline. Obesity Research 1:95S

Hexsel DM, Mazzuco R 2000 Subcision: a treatment for cellulite. International Journal of Dermatology 39:539-544

Jewell ML, Baxter RA, Cox SE, et al 2011 Randomized sham-controlled trial to evaluate the safety and effectiveness of a high-intensity focused ultrasound device for noninvasive body sculpting. Plastic and Reconstructive Surgery 128(1):253-262

Klein KB, Zelickson B, Riopelle JG, et al 2009 Non-invasive cryolipolysis for subcutaneous fat reduction does not affect serum lipid levels or liver function tests. Lasers in Surgery and Medicine 41(10):785-790

Kligman AM, Pagnoni A, Stoudemayer T 1999 Topical retinol improves cellulite. Journal of Dermatologic Treatment 10:119-125

Kulick MI 2010 Evaluation of a noninvasive, dual-wavelength laser-suction and massage device for the regional treatment of cellulite. Plastic and Reconstructive Surgery 125(6): 1788-1796

Lach R 2008 Reduction of subcutaneous fat and improvement in cellulite appearance by dual-wavelength, low-level laser energy combined with vacuum and massage. Journal of Cosmetic and Laser Therapy 10(4):202-209

Manstein D, Laubach H, Watanabe K, et al 2008 Selective cryolysis: a novel method of non-invasive fat removal. Lasers in Surgery and Medicine 40(9):595-604

Mirrashed F, Sharp JC, Krause V, et al 2004 Pilot study of dermal and subcutaneous fat structures by MRI in individuals who differ in gender, BMI, and cellulite grading. Skin Research and Technology 10:161-168

Nootheti PK, Magpantay A, Yosowitz G, et al 2006 A single center, randomized, comparative, prospective clinical study to determine the efficacy of the Velasmooth system versus the Triactive system for the treatment of cellulite. Lasers in Surgery and Medicine 38(10):908-912

Nurnberger F, Muller G 1978 So-called cellulite: an invented disease. Journal of Dermatologic Surgery and Oncology 4:221-229

Pierard-Franchiemont C, Pierand GE, Henry F, et al 2000 A randomized, placebo controlled trial of topical retinal in the treatment of cellulite. American Journal of Clinical Dermatology 1(6):369-374

Querleux B, Cornillon C, Jolivet O 2002 Anatomy and physiology of subcutaneous adipose tissue by in vivo magnetic resonance imaging and spectroscopy: relationships with sex and presence of cellulite. Skin Research and Technology 8:118-124

Rosales-Berber IA, Diliz-Perez E 2009 Controlled cooling of subcutaneous fat for body reshaping. Presented at the 15th World Congress of the International Confederation for Plastic, Reconstructive and Aesthetic Surgery, New Delhi, India

Rossi ABR, Vergnanini AL 2000 Cellulite: a review. Journal of the European Academy of Dermatology and Venereology 14:251-262

Rotunda AM, Avram MM, Avram AS 2005 Cellulite: Is there a role for injectables? Journal of Cosmetic and Laser Therapy 7:147-154

Teitelbaum SA, Burns JL, Kubota J, et al 2007 Noninvasive body contouring by focused ultrasound: safety and efficacy of the Contour I device in a multicenter, controlled, clinical study. Plastic and Reconstructive Surgery 120(3):779-789

Non-surgical skin tightening

9

Melissa A. Bogle, Michael S. Kaminer

Summary and Key Features

- Non-invasive skin tightening is a popular concept with a burgeoning number of devices entering the market

- The main types of non-surgical skin tightening devices include radiofrequency, light, and ultrasound technologies

- Treatment protocols have evolved over the years to focus on reduced energy settings, making the procedures safer and more comfortable for patients

- All skin-tightening devices work by delivering heat in the form of energy to the skin or underlying structures. They create mechanical and biochemical effects that lead to both immediate contraction of collagen fibers and delayed remodeling and neocollagenesis via wound healing

- Patient selection is key for best results and overall patient satisfaction

- Patients who are concerned about risk and recovery and who are willing to accept reduced efficacy in exchange for an improved side effect and healing time profile are ideal candidates for non-ablative approaches

- Non-ablative skin-tightening devices are capable of improving both skin laxity and facial contours. The physician must analyze the patient's three-dimensional facial structure to determine those areas that would benefit most from the procedure. Typically, this would include the upper face/brow region and the lower face/jawline region

- Skin-tightening procedures can be performed along with fillers, neurotoxins or other laser or light-based devices to address multiple issues and achieve a more global overall improvement

- Rarely, patients may experience side effects related to overly aggressive treatment such as burns, indentations, scars or changes in pigmentation. The overall incidence of such problems is extremely low with all current devices owing to updated protocol trends using lower energies and patient feedback as a guide to safe energy delivery

Introduction

The appearance of rhytides and skin laxity are near certainties during the aging process. A number of modalities have been used to reduce the appearance of rhytides and skin laxity, including laser, mechanical, and surgical techniques. Over a decade ago, ablative resurfacing lasers were deemed the gold standard for facial skin tightening. Despite substantial clinical benefits, the technology was beset with significant downtime and an increased risk of side effects such as erythema, permanent pigmentary changes, infection, and scarring. Patients are now more accustomed to procedures with both reduced downtime and sufficient clinical improvement. This has led to a burgeoning number of non-ablative technologies with little to no recovery time and a more favorable risk–reward profile. Unlike ablative lasers, non-ablative technologies induce thermal injury to the dermis or subcutaneous tissues without epidermal vaporization. Epidermal protection is customarily achieved through the use of adjunctive surface cooling.

In terms of skin laxity specifically, the gold standard of treatment remains rhytidectomy or surgical redraping. The goal of this chapter is to review the major types of minimally invasive, non-ablative tissue tightening techniques, including radiofrequency-, light-, and ultrasound-based devices (Table 9.1). These devices are not a replacement for surgical procedures and appropriate patient selection remains key to overall satisfaction.

Thermal collagen remodeling

All skin-tightening devices work by delivering heat in the form of energy to the skin or underlying structures. This creates mechanical and biochemical effects that lead to both immediate contraction of collagen fibers and delayed remodeling and neocollagenesis via a wound-healing response (Box 9.1).

Collagen fibers are composed of a triple helix of protein chains linked with interchain bonds into a crystalline structure. When collagen fibers are heated to specific temperatures, they contract due to breakage of intramolecular hydrogen bonds. Contraction causes the crystalline triple helix structure to fold, creating thicker and shorter collagen fibers. This is thought to be the mechanism of action of immediate tissue tightening seen after skin-tightening

Table 9.1 Major types of skin-tightening technologies

Skin-tightening technology	Device
Monopolar radiofrequency	Thermage® (Solta) Pelleve® (Ellman)
Bipolar radiofrequency with light energy	Galaxy®, Aurora®, Polaris®, ReFirme® (Syneron)
Bipolar radiofrequency with vacuum	Aluma® (Lumenis)
Bipolar radiofrequency delivered via a micro-needle electrode array	ePrime® (Candela-Syneron)
Broadband infrared light	Titan® (Cutera) StarLux IR® (Palomar) SkinTyte® (Sciton)
Unipolar and bipolar radiofrequency	Accent® (Alma)
Ultrasound technology	Ulthera® (Ulthera)

procedures. Studies have also found selective contraction of fibrous septae in the subcutaneous fat, which is thought to be responsible for the inward (Z-dimension) tightening (Fig. 9.1).

Problems can arise if too much heat is delivered as the collagen fibrils will denature completely above a critical heat threshold. This can lead to cell death, denaturation, and scar formation. If too little heat is delivered, there will be no tissue response, although it appears that mild thermal injury gives rise to new dermal ground substance and tissue remodeling of photodamaged skin over time.

> **Box 9.1**
> **Mechanism of skin-tightening devices**
>
> 1. Immediate collagen contraction by direct heating of collagen fibers
> 2. Delayed remodeling and neocollagenesis via a wound-healing response

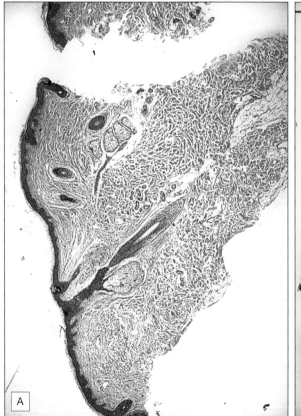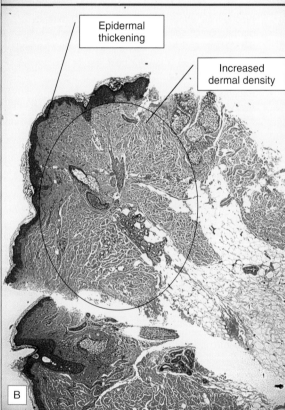

Figure 9.1 Human skin (**A**) before and (**B**) 4 months after treatment with the ThermaCool® TC, showing epidermal thickening and increased dermal density. *Photographs courtesy of Solta.*

Box 9.2
Ohm's law

Impedance (Z) to the movement of electrons creates heat relative to the amount of current (I) and time (t):

$$\text{energy (joules)} = I^2 \times Z \times t$$

Box 9.3
Monopolar electrode devices

- The electrical current passes through a single electrode in the handpiece to a grounding pad
- There is a high density of power close to the electrode's surface with the potential for deep penetration of tissue heating

Box 9.4
Bipolar electrode devices

- The electrical current passes between two electrodes at a fixed distance
- The depth of penetration of the current is limited to approximately one-half the distance between the electrodes

Box 9.5
Factors influencing the depth of penetration of radiofrequency technologies

- Frequency of the electrical current
- Electrode configuration (i.e. monopolar or bipolar)
- Type of tissue serving as the conduction medium
- Temperature

The optimal shrinkage temperature of collagen has been cited as 57–61°C; however, contraction is in actuality determined by a combination of temperature and exposure time. For every 5°C decrease in temperature, a tenfold increase in exposure time is needed to achieve an equivalent amount of collagen contraction. Studies show that for exposure times in the millisecond domain the shrinkage temperature is greater than 85°C, whereas for exposure times over several seconds the shrinkage temperature is at a lower range of 60–65°C.

The other main mechanism in skin rejuvenation is a secondary wound-healing response that produces dermal remodeling over time. The wound-healing response entails activation of fibroblasts to increase deposition of type I collagen and encouraging collagen reorganization into parallel arrays of compact fibrils.

Radiofrequency devices

Radiofrequency devices have been used for hemostasis, electrocoagulation, and endovenous closure in medical dermatology. In the aesthetic arena, the technology has been used for skin resurfacing and non-invasive tissue tightening.

Radiofrequency energy is energy in the electromagnetic spectrum ranging from 300 MHz to 3 kHz. Unlike most lasers, which target specific absorption bands of chromophores, heat is generated from the natural resistance of tissue to the movement of electrons within the radiofrequency field as governed by Ohm's law (Box 9.2). This resistance, called impedance, generates heat relative to the amount of current and time by converting electrical current to thermal energy. Consequently, energy is dispersed to three-dimensional volumes of tissue at controlled depths.

The configuration of electrodes in a radiofrequency device can be monopolar or bipolar, and both have been used for cutaneous applications. The main difference between the two is the configuration of electrodes and type of electromagnetic field that is generated. In a monopolar system, the electrical current passes through a single electrode in the handpiece to a grounding pad (Box 9.3). This type of electrode configuration is common in surgical radiofrequency devices because there is a high density of power close to the electrode's surface with the potential for deep penetration of tissue heating. In tissue-tightening applications, surface cooling is used to protect the outer layers of the skin and heat only deeper targets. In a bipolar system, the electrical current passes between two electrodes at a fixed distance (Box 9.4). This type of electrode configuration has a more controlled current distribution; however, the depth of penetration is limited to approximately one-half the distance between the electrodes.

With radiofrequency technologies, the depth of energy penetration depends upon not only the configuration of the electrodes (i.e. either monopolar or bipolar), but also the type of tissue serving as the conduction medium (i.e. fat, blood, skin), temperature, and the frequency of the electrical current applied (Box 9.5). Tissue is made up of multiple layers, including dermis, fat, muscle, and fibrous tissue, all of which have different resistances to the movement of radiofrequency energy (Table 9.2). Structures with higher impedance are more susceptible to heating. In general, fat, bone, and dry skin tend to have low conductivities such that current tends to flow around these structures rather than through them. Wet skin has a higher electrical conductivity allowing greater penetration of current. This is why, in certain radiofrequency procedures, improved results can be seen with generous amounts of coupling fluid and increased hydration of skin. The structure of each individual's tissue (dermal thickness, fat thickness, fibrous septae, number and size of adnexal structures) all play a role in determining impedance, heat perception, and total deposited energy despite otherwise equal parameters.

Temperature also influences tissue conductivity and the distribution of electrical current. Generally, every 1°C

Table 9.2 Dielectric properties for human tissue at 1 MHz and room temperature

Type of tissue	Electrical conductivity (Siemens/m)
Bone	0.02
Fat	0.03
Dry skin	0.03
Nerve	0.13
Cartilage	0.23
Wet skin	0.22
Muscle	0.50
Thyroid	0.60

increase in temperature lowers the skin impedance by 2%. Surface cooling will increase resistance to the electrical field near the epidermis, driving the radiofrequency current into the tissue and increasing the penetration depth. Conversely, target structures that have been pre-warmed with optical energy will, in theory, have greater conductivity, less resistance, and greater selective heating by the radiofrequency current. This is the theoretical advantage touted by hybrid skin-tightening devices that use a combined approach of light and radiofrequency energy together giving synergistic results.

Monopolar radiofrequency

The first monopolar tissue-tightening device on the market was the ThermaCool® device (Solta Medical, Hayward, CA), introduced in 2001. It remains the most exhaustively studied and published apparatus. The ThermaCool® device uses a capacitive coupled electrode at a single contact point and a high-frequency current at a frequency of 6 MHz. A disposable membrane tip is used to deliver the energy into the skin, with an accompanying adhesive grounding pad serving as a low-resistance path for current flow to complete the circuit. The use of capacitive rather than conductive coupling is important because it allows the energy to be dispersed across a surface to create a zone of tissue heating. With conductive coupling, the energy is concentrated at the tip of the electrode, resulting in increased heating at the contact surface and an increased risk of epidermal injury (Fig. 9.2).

In the early clinical experience, one of the main drawbacks to the ThermaCool® procedure was a high degree of discomfort during the procedure, requiring heavy sedation or frank anesthesia. The protocol at that time was to perform 1–2 passes at higher energies. The treatments were quite painful, results tended to be inconsistent from patient to patient, and some adverse events such as fat necrosis and atrophic scarring were noted. Over the years, treatment protocols have evolved to a paradigm utilizing lower energies, multiple passes, and patient feedback on heat sensation as the end point of therapy. This has all but eliminated the risk of unacceptable side effects and has greatly reduced the pain involved such that most procedures can be performed without any anesthesia. Monopolar radiofrequency energy is now commonly used to accomplish skin tightening of the face, eyelids (Case study 1), abdomen (Fig. 9.3), and extremities.

CASE STUDY 1

A 47-year-old woman presents for a consult regarding excess skin on her upper eyelids. She states she has noticed a gradual increase in drooping over the last several years and she is finding it difficult to wear eye shadow. She has her thirtieth high school reunion in 4 months and states she wants improvement by then. She tells you she is not trying to look 18 again, but just wants to look as good as she feels. On examination, the patient has mild to moderate excess skin laxity on the upper eyelids with minimal bulging of the fat pads. Her brows are in a normal position without significant ptosis. This patient would be a candidate for either radiofrequency skin tightening or a surgical blepharoplasty. She may be a better candidate for non-surgical tightening because of her mild to moderate skin laxity without underlying structural deficits. She also has realistic expectations about results and has several months post-procedure for the skin tightening to take effect before her goal event. Most of the skin-tightening technologies can be used over multiple areas of the body; however, there are a few locations that favor some devices over others. The ThermaCool® device is an excellent choice for skin tightening of eyelid skin because it has a small 0.25 cm² tip, high eye safety profile and lack of significant discomfort during treatment. When the eyelids are being treated, plastic corneoscleral lenses must be put in place. These should be gently inserted and removed so as not to cause erosions of the corneal surface. In addition, the operator should be careful not to deliver too much pressure on the globe, as this can result in vasovagal stimulation and bradycardia. Practitioners should never use ThermaCool® tips larger than the 0.25 cm² eyelid tip owing to the depth of penetration.

Pearl 1

Skin-tightening procedure areas should be carefully inspected post-treatment for signs such as persistent erythema, localized swelling, or hives. If any of these indications are found, it may be helpful to apply a mid- to high-potency topical corticosteroid cream to reduce the incidence of crusting or pigment alteration.

The clinical results of non-ablative radiofrequency skin tightening were first reported by Fitzpatrick and colleagues for the periorbital area in 2003. At least some degree of clinical improvement was reported in 80% of subjects (Figs 9.4–9.6) In 2006, Dover and colleagues

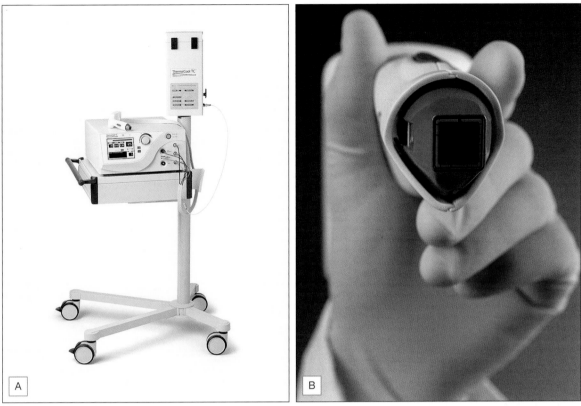

Figure 9.2 (**A**) Thermage ThermaCool® device; (**B**) capacitively coupled electrode treatment tip. *Photographs courtesy of Solta.*

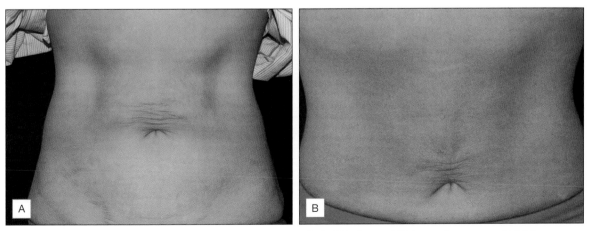

Figure 9.3 Tightening of abdominal skin with the ThermaCool® TC: (**A**) before, and (**B**) 1 year after one pass at 15.5 J.

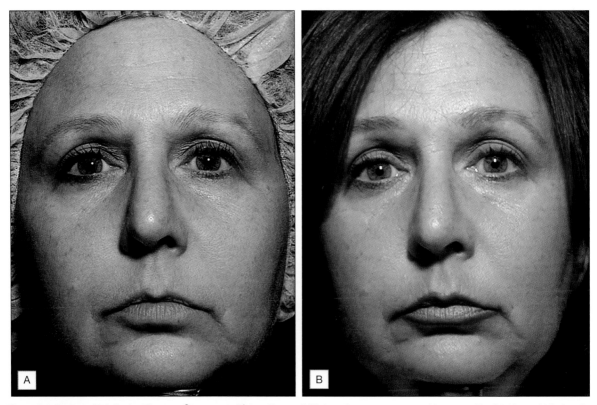

Figure 9.4 Eyebrow lift following Thermage® treatment: (**A**) baseline, and (**B**) 4 weeks post-treatment with a mean lift of 3.42 mm (right brow) and 3.41 mm (left brow). *Photographs courtesy of Solta.*

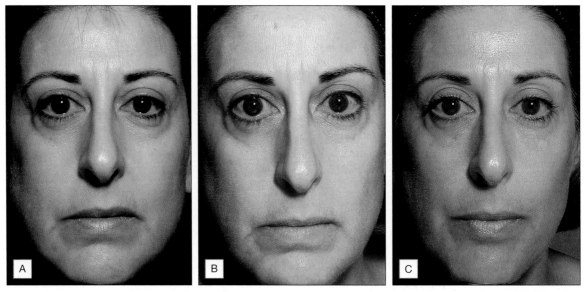

Figure 9.5 Periorbital rejuvenation following Thermage® treatment: (**A**) baseline, (**B**) 2 months post treatment, and (**C**) 4 months post-treatment. *Photographs courtesy of Solta.*

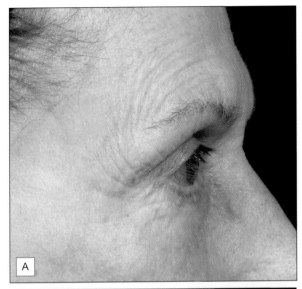

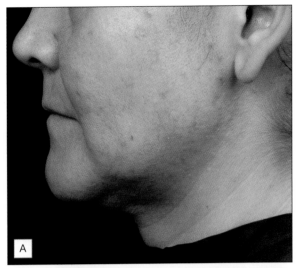

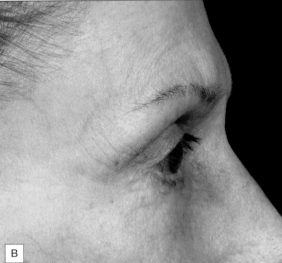

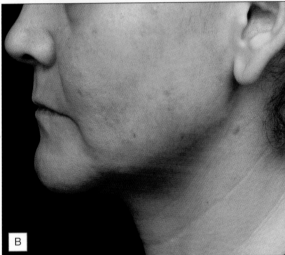

Figure 9.7 Lower-face skin tightening following Thermage®
treatment: (**A**) baseline, and (**B**) 3 months post-treatment.
Photographs courtesy of Dr Ivan Rosales.

Figure 9.6 Periorbital rejuvenation following Thermage® treatment:
(**A**) baseline, and (**B**) 4 months post-treatment. *Photographs courtesy
of Solta Medical Aesthetic Center.*

compared the original single-pass, high-energy technique
with the updated low-energy, multiple-pass technique
using immediate tissue tightening as a real-time end point.
With the original treatment algorithm, 26% of patients
saw immediate tightening, 54% observed skin tightening
at 6 months, and 45% found the procedure overly painful.
With the updated protocol, 87% had immediate tissue
tightening, 92% had some degree of tightening at 6
months, only 5% found the procedure overly painful, and
94% stated the procedure matched their expectations
(Figs 9.7, 9.8). The low-energy, multiple-pass protocol has
also been reported to be significantly safer, lowering the
incidence of adverse events to less than 0.05%.

Pearl 2

Because skin-tightening procedures can cause significant
discomfort, patient pain feedback should be used as the
basis for choosing particular energies in a given treatment
area for each individual. With updated treatment protocols,
anesthesia is usually not required. The use of nerve blocks
and intravenous sedation should not be used as some
degree of pain feedback from the patient is necessary to limit
side effects and enhance patient safety. Local infiltration
anesthesia is also not recommended as it may alter the
inherent tissue impedance and can increase adverse effects.
If in doubt, it is safest to use the lowest possible treatment
settings.

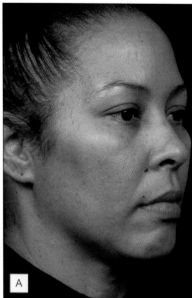

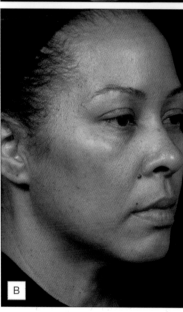

Figure 9.8 Facial skin tightening following Thermage® treatment: (**A**) baseline, and (**B**) 4 months post-treatment. *Photographs courtesy of Solta Medical Aesthetic Center.*

Bipolar radiofrequency

A device using bipolar radiofrequency alone is the ePrime® (Candela-Syneron, Wayland, MA). The ePrime® device is different from other applications on the market in that it uses a microneedle electrode array to deliver bipolar radiofrequency energy into the reticular dermis while bypassing the epidermis and papillary dermis. Single-use treatment cartridges are utilized that contain five independently

controlled, 32-gauge, bipolar microneedle pairs. The 250 μm needles are spaced 1.25 mm apart and each needle pair is independently powered by the generator. The needles are 6 mm long, with the top 3 mm insulated to protect the superficial portion of the skin during treatment, and the bottom 3 mm exposed to allow electrical current flow. The needles are inserted at a 20° angle to the epidermis so that the tip of the needle is 2 mm from the epidermis. Insertion is done by spring-loaded injection. Because current flows between the two needles in each pair, the radiofrequency energy creates five damage zones (one between each pair). If heat is applied long enough, temperature conduction expands the damage zone in all directions. Epidermal cooling is achieved via an integrated thermokinetic cooling bar on the applicator. This approach creates zones of thermal injury with real-time temperature monitoring to help maintain a target temperature of approximately 70°C regardless of varying skin conditions and possibly improve consistency between patients.

Alexiades-Armenakas and colleagues compared baseline and 3–6-month follow-up photographs of 15 patients who underwent skin tightening using a microneedle radiofrequency device with those of 6 patients who had undergone rhytidectomy. The radiofrequency device patients were judged to have a 16% improvement from baseline and the surgical patients were judged to have a 49% improvement from baseline. The authors concluded from this that the mean laxity improvement from a single microneedle radiofrequency treatment was 37% that of a surgical facelift.

Combined electrical and optical energy

Another type of skin-tightening device combines radiofrequency energy with optical energy from laser or light sources. The currently available combined electrical and optical energy devices utilize bipolar electrodes and include the Galaxy®, Aurora®, Polaris®, and ReFirme® systems (Syneron Medical Ltd, Yokneam, Israel). The hypothetical advantage to these devices is that the two forms of energy may act synergistically to generate heat. Target structures that have been pre-warmed with optical energy will, in theory, have greater conductivity, less resistance, and greater selective heating by the radiofrequency current. No grounding pad is required as the current flows between the electrodes rather than throughout the remainder of the body as with monopolar systems. One major adverse event noted with these devices is known as tissue arcing, which can result in tissue burns and possible scar formation. Proper technique will help avoid the issue as arcing has been associated with the handpiece not being properly placed in contact with the skin.

The technology has been used in hair removal, wrinkle reduction, skin tightening, and the treatment of both pigment and vascular disorders (Case study 2). The premise is that less radiofrequency energy is ultimately needed for proper collagen denaturation and remodeling. The major disadvantage to these devices is that bipolar radiofrequency energy does not penetrate very deep into the skin. There is also some criticism that bipolar radiofrequency is unable to produce a uniform, volumetric heating response comparable to monopolar radiofrequency. Furthermore, because the bipolar radiofrequency devices are often combined with other light-based technologies, it is difficult to assess exactly how large a role bipolar radiofrequency plays in the clinical outcomes of such treatments.

CASE STUDY 2

A 54-year-old male presents to your office and states that he has been recently divorced and wants to improve his appearance so that he feels more comfortable re-entering the dating scene. He states he is against injectable treatments such as botulinum toxin or fillers because he does not want to put what he calls 'foreign substances' in his body and he does not want to have to come into the office for repeated maintenance. On examination, he has fair skin with scattered lentigines on the cheeks and forehead and fine telangiectasias over the cheeks and nose creating a blush-type erythema. He has early changes consistent with skin laxity predominantly in the mid-face region, brow, and jawline. Combined electrical and optical energy may be the best option for patients who wish to treat their skin laxity in combination with other signs of photodamage such as lentigines or telangiectasias. A 2002 study by Bitter evaluating a series of 3–5 combined intense pulsed light and radiofrequency energy treatments on photoaged skin revealed a 70% improvement in erythema and telangiectasia, a 78% improvement in lentigines, and a 60% improvement in skin texture as determined by subject satisfaction levels. Because these devices can also be used for hair removal, caution should be used in treating the lower face and neck in a male patient so as not to thin or remove the beard. This patient is fair skinned; however, prudence should also be used when treating darker skin types or tanned skin with devices utilizing an optical component absorbed by pigment. As a general guideline, optical fluences should be lowered by a minimum of 20% when treating darkly pigmented lesions or dense pigment irregularity, even in light-skinned patients, to avoid side effects such as burns, crusting or pigmentary alteration.

Pearl 3

Most skin-tightening treatments using radiofrequency, ultrasound and infrared light are generally safe in all skin types. The exception is technologies that use an optical component absorbed by pigment, such as the intense pulsed light–radiofrequency combination. In these cases, caution should be used when treating Fitzpatrick skin types IV–VI, lighter-skin type patients with a tan, darkly pigmented lesions, or areas of dense pigment irregularity.

In 2005, Doshi & Alster conducted one of the first studies using combined diode and radiofrequency technology with a series of three treatments in 20 female subjects (RF: 50–85 J/cm^2, optical energy: 32–40 J/cm^2). Energy was increased with each session based on the patient's pain tolerance and a clinical response of immediate erythema and edema. Modest improvement was seen in all patients at 3 months; however, improvement was found to be slightly reduced at 6 months. In 2005, Sadick and colleagues conducted a two-center study using combination intense pulsed light and radiofrequency (RF: up to 20 J/cm^2, optical energy: 30–45 J/cm^2) over five treatments for facial rhytides and skin laxity. Modest improvements were reported. Side effects were minimal, but some instances of scarring and crusting occurred. In 2007, Yu and colleagues used combination radiofrequency and infrared energy to study skin tightening in a series of three treatments on 19 female Asian patients (RF: 70–120 J/cm^2, optical energy: 10 J/cm^2). Objective assessment showed mild to moderate improvement in 26–47% of areas treated (Figs 9.9, 9.10).

Vacuum-assisted bipolar radiofrequency

Bipolar radiofrequency has been combined with an accompanying vacuum apparatus in an attempt to take advantage of several benefits of vacuum technology. The first device to do this was the Aluma® (Lumenis, Santa Clara, CA) using what has been termed FACES (functional aspiration controlled electrothermal stimulation) technology. The vacuum apparatus suctions a fold of skin in alignment between two electrodes. Non-target structures such as muscle, fascia, and bone are avoided. The theory is that this may help to overcome the depth limitations inherent in bipolar radiofrequency technology by bringing the target tissue closer to the electrodes. Less overall energy may also be required for an effective treatment. It has also been hypothesized that increased blood flow and mechanical stress of fibroblasts from the vacuum suction may lead to increased collagen formation. Vacuum technology has the added benefit of helping to reduce procedure discomfort.

In a pilot study of 46 adults undergoing eight facial treatments with vacuum-assisted bipolar radiofrequency, Gold found significant improvements in skin texture. The mean elastosis score of study participants went from 4.5 pre-treatment to 2.5 by 6 months post-treatment, indicating a shift from moderate to mild elastosis. The authors noted a short-term tightening effect due to collagen contraction followed by a gradual, long-term improvement due to the wound-healing response and neocollagenesis. Although subjects were generally pleased with the treatment outcome, their satisfaction levels declined somewhat during the follow-up period. This can be a common finding in radiofrequency skin treatments owing to delayed neocollagenesis and long-term wound-healing response. Subjects may have difficulty accurately remembering the exact condition of their skin pre-treatment, particularly when 6 or more months have passed.

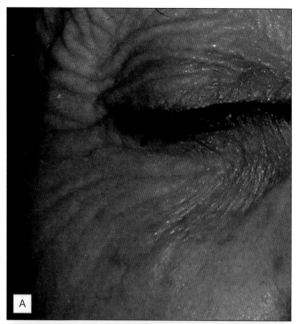

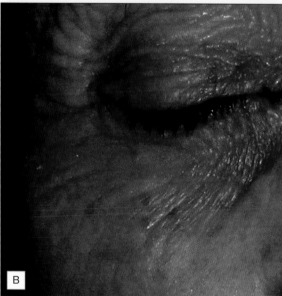

Figure 9.9 Periorbital rejuvenation: (**A**) before, and (**B**) after three treatments with the Galaxy® device.

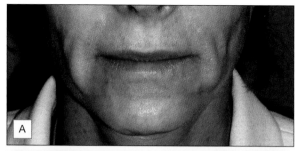

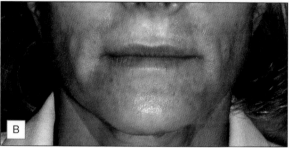

Figure 9.10 Lower-face skin tightening: (**A**) before, and (**B**) immediately following a single treatment with the Galaxy® device.

Hybrid monopolar and bipolar radiofrequency

The first system to combine monopolar and bipolar radio-frequency in one device was the Accent® (Alma Lasers, Buffalo Grove, IL). The theory behind using both types of radiofrequency is to deliver different depths of current to the skin. The bipolar electrode handpiece allows for more superficial, localized (non-volumetric) heating based on tissue resistance to the radiofrequency conductive current. The monopolar electrode handpiece targets deeper, volumetric heating via the rotational movement of water molecules in the alternating current of the electromagnetic field. The monopolar handpiece delivers a higher amount of energy since it theoretically is heating a greater tissue volume than the bipolar handpiece. Typically the monopolar handpiece is used to treat the forehead, cheeks, jawline, and neck (Fig. 9.11). The bipolar handpiece is used to treat the glabella, lateral periorbital area (Fig. 9.12), upper lip and chin, and leg (Fig. 9.13). Despite the use of monopolar radiofrequency, this particular system uses a closed system where no grounding plate is required (Case study 3).

CASE STUDY 3

A 42-year-old woman comes into your office with the complaint of skin laxity in the upper arm area. She states she is no longer comfortable wearing sleeveless clothing because she feels like her arms look like what she calls 'cottage cheese'. She states she has always maintained a relatively normal weight. On examination, she is of a normal weight for

Pearl 4

It is essential to take standardized photographs before skin-tightening procedures. Care should be taken to use identical positioning and lighting conditions in all photography sessions, as subtle differences can distort appearance and alter perceived outcomes. Pre-treatment and post-treatment photographs may need to be compared since changes with skin-tightening procedures may be subtle to the patient, especially after several months have passed.

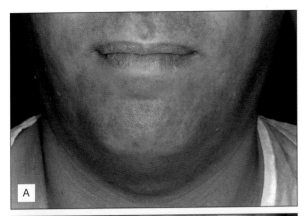

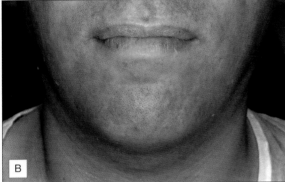

Figure 9.11 Skin tightening of the neck and jawline region: (**A**) before, and (**B**) immediately following a single treatment with the Accent® treatment. *Photographs courtesy of Dr Alexiades-Armenakas.*

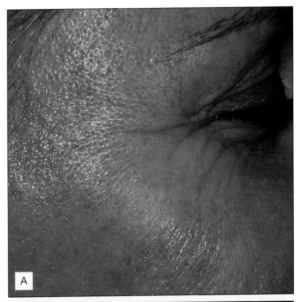

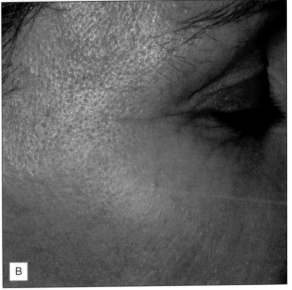

Figure 9.12 Periorbital rejuvenation: (**A**) before, and (**B**) 3 months after four treatments with the Accent® treatment. *Photographs courtesy of Dr Alexiades-Armenakas.*

her height and build. She has a mild to moderate skin laxity predominantly in the posterior portion of her upper arm and dimpling in the texture of both the anterior and posterior surface of the arms. In this case the patient has two main options for improvement including upper arm liposuction and non-surgical skin tightening. She may be a better candidate for non-surgical skin tightening because the textural abnormality in her upper arms extends around the full circumference. Liposuction would predominantly improve the skin in the 'bat wing' area on the posterior portion of the arm. She would not be a candidate for surgical brachioplasty due to her young age, milder degree of laxity, and desire to wear sleeveless clothing. In this case, the hybrid Accent® device would be a good choice for tissue tightening with the added benefit of possible volume reduction. One case report compared treating skin laxity on one arm with the ThermaCool® device and the opposite arm with the Accent® device. The ThermaCool® arm was treated with a single treatment at settings of 351.5–354 with a minimum of six passes on the inner arm and three passes on the outer arm (1200 pulses total). The Accent® arm was treated with a series of nine treatments at 2-week intervals using the monopolar handpiece at an epidermal temperature of 42.5°C with three therapeutic phase passes. Although skin texture improved with both

treatments, the Accent®-treated arm was reported to be tighter and firmer after just two treatments, with a looser-fitting clothing sleeve. Because the ThermaCool®-treated arm did not have a looser fitting clothing sleeve until the physician had gone back at the end of the study and performed two Accent® treatments, the author suggested that the Accent® radiofrequency energy penetrates deeper and may be the device of choice when patients require both tissue tightening and volume reduction.

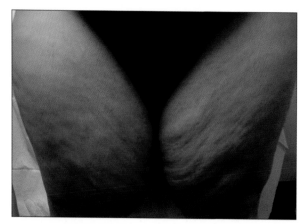

Figure 9.13 Cellulite treatment on the right leg following five treatments with the Accent® and the left leg serving as an untreated control. *Photograph courtesy of Dr Alexiades-Armenakas.*

In 2007, Friedman treated 16 patients with a hybrid monopolar and bipolar radiofrequency device; 56% of participants had at least some degree of improvement in the appearance of rhytides and skin laxity. Twelve patients had cheek treatments, with 5 achieving 51–75% improvement and 2 achieving greater than 75% improvement. Nine had jowl treatments, with 4 achieving 51–75% improvement and 1 achieving greater than 75% improvement. Younger patients (25–45 years of age) were found to have a higher satisfaction rate than older patients.

Pearl 5

Studies suggest that younger patients may respond better than older patients. This may be because heat-labile collagen bonds are progressively replaced by irreducible multivalent cross-links as the tissue ages, such that the skin of older individuals is less amenable to heat-induced tissue tightening. Skin quality is more important than absolute age of the patient. Older patients with relatively good skin quality can respond just as well as their younger counterparts.

The Pelleve® device (Ellman International, Oceanside, NY) has taken advantage of a dual monopolar and bipolar radiofrequency-based surgical unit normally used for tissue cutting and coagulation to make it suitable for skin-tightening procedures. The system works with the use of reusable probes that are plugged into the system and applied over the skin in a circular pattern to heat the subdermal tissue. A chilled coupling gel is used to assure proper coupling between the electrode and the patient and to help protect the epidermis. As with other skin-tightening devices, the gentle heating induces collagen denaturation, contraction, and subsequent synthesis. Repeat treatments have been shown to improve the appearance of wrinkles and skin laxity, but results are somewhat limited due to the discrete amount of energy applied. Early protocols recommended 8-weekly treatments for best results, but the treatment paradigm has since been revised to two treatments spaced 1 month apart, with some patients requiring an additional treatment.

Infrared light devices

Broadband infrared light in the range of 800 to 1800 nm, depending on the device, has been utilized for non-ablative tissue tightening. The infrared rays are selectively filtered to achieve gradual heating of the dermis, with pre, parallel, and post-cooling to assure epidermal protection. The first such light-based system on the market was the Titan® (Cutera, Brisbane, CA). It utilizes light energy in the range of 1100 to 1800 nm to target water as a chromophore, causing collagen denaturation and ultimately collagen remodeling and tissue tightening. The StarLux IR® (Palomar Medical Technologies, Burlington, MA) delivers fractionated energy through the handpiece of the device at a wavelength range of 850 to 1350 nm, which also targets water as the principal chromophore. Multiple treatments are required for optimal results. The SkinTyte® device (Sciton, Palo Alto, CA) utilizes light at a wavelength range of 800 to 1400 nm.

In 2006, Ruiz-Esparza performed one to three treatments on 25 patients utilizing broadband infrared light from 1100 to 1800 nm. Most patients showed improvement ranging from minimal to excellent with immediate skin tightening visible in 22 of the 25 patients. Three patients showed no improvement. The best results were achieved when using a combination of lower fluences and a high number of pulses. Patients treated at 30 J/cm² expressed no pain during the procedure and had a high degree of satisfaction immediately post-procedure. The same year, Zelickson and colleagues looked at ultrastructural changes in cadaver and human skin post-treatment. Collagen fibril alteration was found to be highest with greater fluences and depths of 1–2 mm. Marginal results were observed at shallower depths and lower fluences, which were possibly due to the effect of contact cooling. Comparison of the two studies emphasizes that clinical skin tightening does not always correlate with immediate positive histological findings. This is explained by the fact that full clinical effect may take weeks or months to be demonstrated owing to a secondary wound healing response.

In 2006, a multi-center study reported longer-term (12–18-month) results using the 1100–1800 nm infrared device at 34–36 J/cm². Results were both immediate and delayed up to 6 months. Clinical outcomes ranged from mild to moderate in most patients. The authors concluded that using a lower fluence range of 30–40 J/cm², 2–3 treatments, 1–2 passes, and extra passes on areas that need immediate contraction or along vector lines yielded best results.

When treating the face, the physician should look at the face as distinct regions. Although the entire face can be treated in one session, it is also possible to treat segmental areas alone such as the forehead, the eyelids, or the cheek/jawline region. However, treatment of broader surface areas and treatment of areas adjacent to the described area of laxity may improve results.

Complications were limited to minor erythema, but a few blisters were observed in areas that were overtreated. In 2007, Goldberg and colleagues noted positive results in 11 of 12 patients receiving two treatments with the same device (30–36 J/cm²). The best results were observed in patients who had loose draping skin, with less significant results in sagging skin that was firmly associated with the subcutaneous tissue. No improvement was noted in the jowl region.

Non-surgical skin tightening is best suited to patients with mild to moderate skin laxity without significant underlying structural ptosis. Patients with underlying structural laxity, including that of the facial musculature or superficial muscular aponeurotic system (SMAS), and patients with an excessive amount of skin laxity are likely to have limited or no improvement and should be counseled on other methods of rejuvenation including surgery.

Other laser wavelengths that have been used for tissue tightening include the 1064 nm and 1320 nm wavelengths. The chromophores for the 1064 nm wavelength, in decreasing order, are melanin, hemoglobin and water, and the primary chromophore for the 1320 nm wavelength is water. A 2005 study by Taylor & Prokopenko compared a single treatment using a monopolar radiofrequency system (73.5 J/cm²) with a single treatment using the 1064 nm neodymium:yttrium-aluminum-garnet (Nd:YAG) laser (50 J/cm²). The 1064 nm laser side was deemed to have better overall results in terms of improvement in wrinkles and skin laxity, although only modest improvements was noted in both modalities. Another study in 2007 by Key compared a single facial treatment with a monopolar radiofrequency system (40 J/cm²) to the 1064 nm Nd:YAG laser (73–79 J/cm²). The 1064 nm laser resulted in greater improvement on the lower face, while improvement on the upper face was equivalent with both modalities. In 2001, Trelles and colleagues treated 10 patients with a series of eight treatments using a 1320 nm laser system (30–35 J/cm²). Clinical improvement was subtle, with only two patients reporting satisfaction with the procedure. The authors suggested combining laser treatment with parallel epidermal treatment may yield better results and achieve higher patient satisfaction.

Combination therapy is a leading theme in cosmetic dermatology. Patients are able to achieve a better overall result when procedures such as non-surgical skin tightening are combined with other therapies such as botulinum toxin, fillers, and other modalities. For example, patients desiring a brow lift and a more defined jawline may achieve benefit from the use of botulinum toxin to the superior-lateral orbicularis oculi and platysma muscles in addition to skin tightening. Fillers can be used to achieve additional lift in the mid face, brow/temples, pre-jowl region, and jawline.

Ultrasound devices

High-intensity focused ultrasound (HIFU) is the most recent player to enter the skin-tightening technology realm. When an intense ultrasound field vibrates tissue, friction is created between molecules causing them to absorb mechanical energy and leading to secondary generation of heat. Thus, the primary mechanism responsible for tissue necrosis with focused ultrasound treatment is heating of the tissue due to the absorption of acoustic energy. Ideally, this leads to immediate tissue contraction and delayed collagen remodeling with the coagulative change limited to the focal region of the ultrasound field. In reality, the spectrum of cellular changes depends on the rise in temperature and the exposure duration and can range from total necrosis to subtler ultrastructural cell damage with modulation of cellular cytokine expression.

Intense focused ultrasound for skin-tightening applications uses short, millisecond pulses with a frequency in the megahertz (MHz) domain, rather than kilohertz (kHz) as is used in traditional HIFU, to avoid cavitational processes. Intense focused ultrasound also uses significantly lower energies than traditional HIFU, 0.5–10 J versus 100 J, which allows thermal tissue changes without gross necrosis. The main advantage to focused ultrasound is the potential for greater depth of skin changes than other technologies with the added benefit of precisely controlled, focal tissue injury. Ultrasound energy is able to target deeper structures in a select, focused fashion without secondary scatter and absorption in the dermis and epidermis. Early research on human cadaveric tissue showed intense ultrasound energy was able to target the facial superficial musculo-aponeurotic system (SMAS) to produce discrete zones of thermal injury while sparing non-targeted adjacent structures.

The first intense focused ultrasound device on the market is the Ulthera® system (Ulthera Inc., Mesa, AZ). The system incorporates ultrasound imaging capability for visualizing the skin and deep tissue in combination with a therapeutic ultrasound module that creates small, approximately 1 mm³, wedge-shaped zones of thermal coagulation. The thermally induced zones result from selective absorption of ultrasound energy in the area of geometric focus of the beam. The depth and volume of the thermal lesions are determined by the preset focus depth and frequency of the probe in combination with the intrinsic characteristics of the tissue being treated. The source energy is an adjustable parameter. Higher-frequency probes are associated with more superficial tissue effect whereas lower-frequency probes are associated with a deeper tissue effect. Typically, higher-frequency probes are used to treat areas of thinner skin such as that of the neck, whereas the lower-frequency probes are used to treat areas of thicker skin such as that of the cheeks.

Current protocols aim for a geometric focal depth of therapy in the mid to deep dermis. One of the first clinical trials by Alam and colleagues in 2010 assessed the safety and efficacy of intense focused ultrasound on skin tightening. Significant improvement was seen in brow elevation in more than 83% of treated patients with an average increase in brow elevation of 1.7–1.9 mm (Fig. 9.14). Results developed over a 90-day period following treatment and were still noticeable at 10-month follow-up. The authors found lower face tightening more difficult to assess due to a lack of fixed anatomical landmarks. In 2011, Suh and colleagues treated 22 Asian patients with

facial skin laxity with intense focused ultrasound; 77% of patients reported much improvement in the nasolabial folds, and 73% reported much improvement in the jaw line. Histological evaluation of skin samples showed greater dermal collagen with thickening of the dermis and straightening of elastic fibers in the reticular dermis after treatment (Figs 9.15 and 9.16).

Due to the relatively recent development of the device, large-scale trials are lacking and optimal treatment protocols are still being developed. Temporary nerve side effects can occur. Future advances may fine tune even deeper

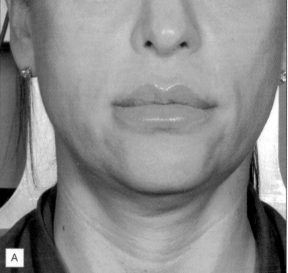

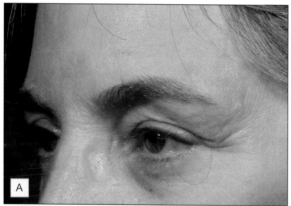

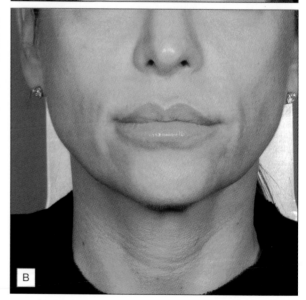

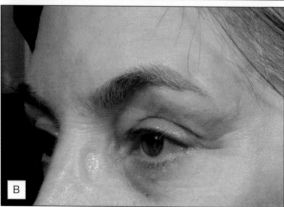

Figure 9.14 Periorbital rejuvenation and brow lift following Ultherapy® treatment: (**A**) baseline, and (**B**) post single-depth treatment using the 3.0 mm transducer or 4.5 mm transducer depth based on the periorbital region. *Photographs courtesy of Dr Jeff Dover.*

Figure 9.15 Lower-face skin tightening following Ultherapy® treatment: (**A**) baseline, and (**B**) post dual-depth treatment at 3.0 mm and 4.5 mm depths. *Photographs courtesy of Ulthera Inc.*

and occur over a period of 3–6 months. In terms of expectations, these technologies should not be thought of as an equivalent technology to surgical lifting, but as an alternative option for a certain subset of patients. Despite a number of clinical studies reporting significant improvement in the appearance of lax skin, most patients show only mild improvement. It appears that patients who are younger with a lesser degree of skin laxity may yield the most promising clinical outcomes; skin laxity without a significant muscular attachment also appears to yield better results (Case study 4). Very elderly patients with severe sagging and wrinkles are, in general, suboptimal candidates for the degree of improvement expected with non-invasive tightening devices (Case study 5).

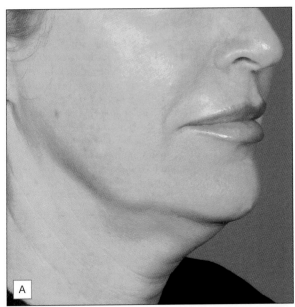

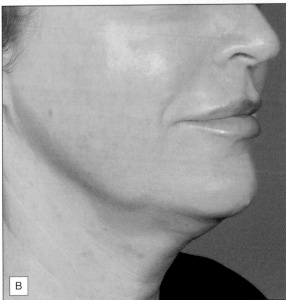

Figure 9.16 Lower-face skin tightening following Ultherapy® treatment: (**A**) baseline, and (**B**) post dual-depth treatment at 3.0 mm and 4.5 mm depths. *Photographs courtesy of Ulthera Inc.*

delivery of energy with the goal of producing focused thermal collagen denaturation in the SMAS.

Tips for maximizing patient satisfaction

Patient selection is of utmost importance in ultimate satisfaction with non-surgical skin-tightening technologies. Patients must be counseled that maximum results are slow

CASE STUDY 4

A 78-year-old woman presents for a consult regarding general photoaging. She has avoided sun exposure her whole life and is a devoted wearer of sunscreen. She tells you she has been going to an esthetician for the past 15 years who gives her light glycolic peels every few months. She has also used a prescription tretinoin cream given to her by her general dermatologist for the past 25 years. She is otherwise healthy and would like to improve her appearance, but she would like to get your advice on what she needs. She has never had surgery before and tells you she would like to avoid having a facelift if possible. On examination she has remarkably preserved skin quality with very few deep lines and no major pigmentary issues owing to her diligent sun protection and long-term use of topical rejuvenation therapies. She does have some loss of definition along the jawline, with mild to moderate jowling, deepening of the nasolabial folds, descent of the eyebrow, and volume-related changes in the mid-face region. She also has prominent platysmal banding visible in the neck region. This patient would be an ideal candidate for almost any of the non-invasive skin-tightening approaches in combination with other therapies such as neurotoxins and fillers to augment her results. Although studies have shown that younger patients tend to have better results than older patients after tissue tightening procedures, this patient has extremely good skin quality and can be expected to have at least some degree of improvement. Because the skin-tightening procedure will not address her underlying changes in facial volume and musculature, performing adjunctive therapies such as botulinum toxin to the superior-lateral orbicularis oculi and platysma muscles would help her lift the brow, decrease banding on the neck, and achieve a more defined jawline. Filler to her mid-face region, nasolabial folds, pre-jowl region, and jawline would also be of use to restore underlying structure, increase the lifting effect, and give a more youthful shape to the face. A 2006 study by Shumaker and colleagues showed monopolar radiofrequency skin tightening to be safe when performed over multiple soft tissue fillers and indicated it may even have some synergistic effects in terms of long-term collagen growth. The patient has proven she is not averse to maintenance therapies and she will achieve a better overall result with global rejuvenation.

CASE STUDY 5

A 66-year-old year old woman comes to your office to discuss options regarding skin laxity on the face. She states she has always loved the sun and shares tales of her days lying out on her roof with a foil blanket, covered in baby oil and iodine. She states she does not purposely tan anymore, but her husband loves to play golf and go boating. She normally accompanies him, but she has not been able to since she was diagnosed with an irregular heart rhythm last year and her cardiologist implanted a pacemaker. During the consultation, she pulls her facial skin back tautly with her hands and tells you her wrinkles do not bother her, but she would be happy if she could get rid of her sagging skin. On examination, the patient has a thin body habitus with severe solar elastosis and significant skin laxity. This is a difficult patient clinically because she is not a good candidate for non-surgical skin tightening for several reasons. The first issue is her pacemaker device. Radiofrequency treatments are contraindicated in patients with pacemakers, internal defibrillators, or metal implants on the face. This also makes her an undesirable candidate for a surgical facelift. Although she could undergo non-surgical skin tightening with one of the broadband infrared light devices, she has very poor skin quality and a considerable degree of laxity. This, combined with her desire for facelift-like results, would most likely lead to disappointment after the procedure.

Patients should be told that non-ablative skin tightening is not a substitute for a facelift and that results may be modest (Box 9.6). A small number of patients perceive no improvement at all. Patients should also be counseled that non-ablative skin tightening alone is not effective for the textural aspects of photoaging including wrinkles and pigmentary alterations. Long-term studies to examine the longevity of skin tightening have not been performed, but it appears patients can expect at least a period of a year or more before touch-up treatments are required. More research also needs to be done comparing the devices themselves to determine precise advantages of one over another.

Conclusion

The quest for non-surgical skin tightening has led to a burgeoning number of devices on the market. Although dermal remodeling may occur with radiofrequency-, optical-, and ultrasound-based devices, patients and physicians should not expect results to be similar to those seen after surgical or possibly even ablative techniques. The techniques appear best suited for younger patients with mild to moderate skin laxity without a significant degree of underlying structural ptosis. Physicians must appreciate the indications, complications, benefits, and limitations of each device. The key to success remains rooted in patient selection and management of expectations. It is still uncertain as to how many treatments are ideal for the majority of these medical devices and how long the effects will be maintained. Future research and clinical trials will continue to refine techniques and delivery systems for optimal results.

Further reading

Alam M, White L, Martin N, et al 2010 Ultrasound tightening of facial and neck skin: A rater-blinded prospective cohort study. Journal of the American Academy of Dermatology 62:262-269

Alexiades-Armenakas M, Rosenberg D, Renton B, et al 2010 Blinded, randomized, quantitative grading comparison of minimally invasive, fractional radiofrequency and surgical face-lift to treat skin laxity. Archives of Dermatology 146:396-405

Atiyeh BS, Dibo SA 2009 Nonsurgical nonablative treatment of aging skin: radiofrequency technologies between aggressive marketing and evidence-based efficacy. Aesthetic Plastic Surgery 33:283-294

Biesman BS, Pope K 2007 Monopolar radiofrequency treatment of the eyelids: a safety evaluation. Dermatologic Surgery 33:794-801

Bitter P Jr, Mulholland RS 2002 Report of a new technique for enhanced non-invasive skin rejuvenation using a dual mode pulsed light and radiofrequency energy source: selective radiothermolysis. Journal of Cosmetic Dermatology 1:142-145

Doshi SN, Alster TS 2005 Combined diode laser and RF energy for rhytides and skin laxity: investigation of a novel device. Journal of Cosmetic and Laser Therapy 7:11-15

Dover JS, Zelickson B, and the 14-Physician multispecialty consensus panel 2007 Results of a survey of 5,700 patient monopolar radiofrequency facial skin tightening treatments: assessment of a low-energy multiple-pass technique leading to a clinical end point algorithm. Dermatologic Surgery 33:900-907

Fitzpatrick R, Geronemus R, Goldberg D, et al 2003 Multicenter study of noninvasive radiofrequency for periorbital tissue tightening. Lasers in Surgery and Medicine 33:232-242

Friedman DJ, Gilead LT 2007 The use of hybrid radiofrequency device for the treatment of rhytides and lax skin. Dermatologic Surgery 33:543-551

Gold MH 2010 Update on tissue tightening. Journal of Clinical and Aesthetic Dermatology 3:36-41

Gold MH, Goldman MP, Rao J, et al 2007 Treatment of wrinkles and elastosis using vacuum-assisted bipolar radiofrequency heating of the dermis. Dermatologic Surgery 33:300-309

Goldberg DJ, Hussain M, Fazeli A, et al 2007 Treatment of skin laxity of the lower face and neck in older individuals with a broad-spectrum infrared light device. Journal of Cosmetic and Laser Therapy 9:35-40

Hantash BM, Renton B, Berkowitz RL, et al 2009 Pilot clinical study of a novel minimally invasive bipolar microneedle radiofrequency device. Lasers in Surgery and Medicine 41:87-95

Hsu TS, Kaminer MS 2003 The use of nonablative radiofrequency technology to tighten the lower face and neck. Seminars in Cutaneous Medicine and Surgery 22:115-123

Key DJ 2007 Single-treatment skin tightening by RF and long-pulsed, 1064-nm Nd:YAG laser compared. Lasers in Surgery and Medicine 2:169-175

Laubach HJ, Makin IR, Barthe PG, et al 2008 Intense focused ultrasound: evaluation of a new treatment modality for precise microcoagulation within the skin. Dermatologic Surgery 34:727-734

Mayoral FA 2007 Skin tightening with a combined unipolar and bipolar radiofrequency device. Journal of Drugs in Dermatology 6:212-215

Narins RS, Tope WD, Pope K, et al 2006 Overtreatment effects associated with a radiofrequency tissue-tightening device: rare, preventable, and correctable with subcision and autologous fat transfer. Dermatologic Surgery 32:115-124

Ruiz-Esparza J 2006 Painless, nonablative, immediate skin contraction induced by low-fluence irradiation with new infrared device: a report of 25 patients. Dermatologic Surgery 32:60-610

Sadick NS, Alexiades-Armenakas M, Bitter P Jr, et al 2005 Enhanced full-face skin rejuvenation using synchronous intense pulsed optical and conducted bipolar RF energy (ELOS): Introducing selective radiophotothermolysis. Journal of the European Academy of Dermatology and Venereology 4:181-186

Sadick NS, Shaoul J 2004 Hair removal using a combination of conducted radiofrequency and optical energies – an 18-month follow-up. Journal of Cosmetic and Laser Therapy 6:21-26

Shumaker PR, England LJ, Dover JS, et al 2006 Effect of monopolar radiofrequency treatment over soft-tissue fillers in an animal model: Part 2. Lasers in Surgery and Medicine 38:211-217

Suh DH, Shin MK, Lee SJ, et al 2011 Intense focused ultrasound tightening in Asian skin: clinical and pathologic results. Dermatologic Surgery 37(11):1595-1602

Taub AF, Battle EF Jr, Nikolaidis G 2006 Multicenter clinical perspectives on a broadband infrared light device for skin tightening. Journal of Drugs in Dermatology 5(8):771-778

Taylor MB, Prokopenko I 2006 Split-face comparison of RF versus long-pulse Nd:YAG treatment of facial laxity. Journal of Cosmetic and Laser Therapy 8:17-22

Trelles MA, Allones I, Luna R 2001 Facial rejuvenation with a nonablative 1320-nm Nd:YAG laser: a preliminary clinical and histologic evaluation. Dermatologic Surgery 27:111-116

Yu CS, Yeung CK, Shek SY, et al 2007 Combined infrared light and bipolar RF for skin tightening in Asians. Lasers in Surgery and Medicine 39:471-475

Zelickson B, Ross V, Kist D, et al 2006 Ultrastructural effects of an infrared handpiece on forehead and abdominal skin. Dermatologic Surgery 32:897-901

10

Laser treatment of ethnic skin

Stephanie G.Y. Ho, Henry H.L. Chan

Summary and Key Features

- The use of lasers and lights can be safe and effective in ethnic skin

- Sun protection pre- and post-treatment, together with the use of bleaching agents, is important in reducing the risks of post inflammatory hyperpigmentation

- Q-switched and long pulsed lasers are both useful in the treatment of epidermal pigmentation; however, in ethnic skin, long-pulsed lasers are preferred as they have similar efficacy with less side effects

- Using a small spot size avoids inadvertent treatment of surrounding normal skin, which can increase the risk of hyperpigmentation when the contrast between lesional and non-lesional skin is low

- Diascopy during treatment of pigmented lesions reduces the risk of vascular damage

- Longer wavelength lasers allow for dermal pigmentation to be treated

- Q-switched 1064 nm Nd:YAG laser, in conjunction with 1550 nm fractional resurfacing, can achieve optimal results in the treatment of nevus of Ota

- Hori's macules can be resistant to treatment, requiring multiple treatments. There is also a risk of initial darkening of pigmentation before subsequent lightening with further treatments

- Melasma is a common pigmentary condition in ethnic skin and a challenge to treat. Topical bleaching agents should be used before laser therapy is considered

- Non-ablative fractional resurfacing using lower densities but increasing the number of treatment sessions is recommended for ethnic skin

Introduction

The evolution of population demographics in the 21st century is such that patients with ethnic skin will become of increasing importance to any practicing dermatologist.

Ethnic skin comprises a diverse group, including Chinese, Japanese, Indian, Pakistani, Hispanic, Latino, African, Afro-Caribbean, and African American. Their skin color typically falls within the Fitzpatrick's skin phototypes III–VI.

Ethnic skin differs from the Caucasian counterpart in several aspects. The larger melanocytes in skin of color produce more melanin and melanosomes are distributed individually in keratinocytes, conferring significant photoprotection. Photoaging tends to manifest more frequently as pigmentary changes, as opposed to wrinkle formation. Congenital and acquired pigmentary disorders such as nevus of Ota, Hori's macules, and melasma are also more commonly encountered. Management of pigmentary conditions is therefore an important concern for most patients with ethnic skin. However, the high melanin content in such skin, coupled with the broad absorption of melanin on the electromagnetic spectrum, can often present therapeutic challenges during laser treatment, as a competing chromophore to the intended pigmented target is present throughout ethnic skin. Post-inflammatory hyperpigmentation (PIH), rarely seen in light-colored skin, can be a common outcome during inexperienced laser use in darker skin types. This chapter aims to discuss the effective and safe use of laser and light sources in the management of common conditions seen in ethnic skin, in order to optimize results and minimize complications. We will also highlight good practices to adopt, and pitfalls to avoid.

Evaluating the patient with ethnic skin

A thorough history and examination are essential in establishing a correct diagnosis prior to treatment. Standardized digital photography is helpful in recording the baseline appearance, and any subsequent improvement. Additional aids such as UV photography or Wood's light can be useful, for example, in assessing the epidermal and dermal components of melasma. The patient's treatment objective and expectation should be enquired, and treatment options and associated risks discussed. Providing additional printed material regarding suggested procedures is often helpful. Obtaining informed consent prior to procedure is essential and good practice. Establishing realistic patient expectations through good rapport is imperative in achieving a satisfactory outcome.

A detailed patient interview can identify the patient's concern and highlight the primary problem, which must be addressed. For example, a patient presenting for management of acne PIH and scarring will require treatment for their active acne before embarking on treatment of the secondary complications. Any relative contraindications to laser and light treatment should be excluded, such as infection or recent sun exposure of the treatment site, isotretinoin use in the last 6 months, photosensitivity or use of photosensitizing drugs, immunocompromised state, predisposition towards keloid or hypertrophic scarring, pregnancy, and personal or family history of melanoma. The patient's Fitzpatrick's skin type should be noted.

Taking a thorough medical history also helps clinicians identify patients who have unrealistic expectations, or psychiatric disorders such as body dysmorphic disorders (BDD). Such patients have an excessive preoccupation with an imagined or slight defect in appearance, which results in a clinically significant distress and impairment in functioning. A recent study reviewing 401 adults with BDD symptoms in an ethnically diverse group found significant differences between Asians and Caucasians, with Asians reporting more concerns with straight hair and dark skin, and less concerns about body shape. A simple and reliable questionnaire for the diagnosis of BDD has been developed by Dufresne and colleagues, and can be a useful adjunct in suspected cases. BDD is a contraindication to laser treatments, and these patients should be referred for psychiatric and psychotherapeutic treatments.

Obtaining written consent with a clear outline of risks and benefits is essential and protects both the clinician and the patient. The clinician should ensure that patients have a good understanding of different treatment options, the expected outcome, the associated downtime, postoperative care, and potential risks from the procedure. There should be adequate opportunity for the patient to have all their questions answered.

Any sun exposure during several weeks prior to laser treatment can predispose patients with ethnic skin to a higher risk of post-inflammatory hyper or hypopigmentation. The use of sunscreens and topical bleaching agents for at least 2 weeks prior to any such treatment can help reduce the risk of PIH. Patients should be provided written guidance regarding postoperative care, with additional emphasis on sun protection and avoidance for at least 4 weeks after.

Treatment of epidermal pigmentation

Freckles and lentigines

Freckles and lentigines are benign pigmented lesions commonly seen in ethnic skin. Freckles occur in adolescence and are relatively uniform in distribution, size and color. Histologically, they are characterized by epidermal hypermelanosis without an increase in melanocyte numbers. Lentigines tend to appear later and vary in size, color and distribution. Histologically, both epidermal

hypermelanosis and increase in melanocyte numbers are seen. Epidermal rete ridges are also elongated and clubbed.

As melanin has a broad absorption spectrum ranging from 250 to 1200 nm, various lasers have been used to target cutaneous pigmentation, usually with excellent results. Anderson et al were the first to demonstrate the effectiveness of Q-switched (QS) lasers in the treatment of cutaneous pigmentation. Frequency-doubled QS neodymium:yttrium-aluminum-garnet (Nd:YAG), QS ruby, and QS alexandrite lasers with respective wavelengths of 532 nm, 694 nm, and 755 nm, have all been used with good results in lighter-skinned patients but PIH risk of 10–25% has been reported when used on ethnic skin. Chan et al compared 532 nm frequency-doubled Nd:YAG lasers with different pulse durations in the treatment of facial lentigines in Chinese patients, and found similar efficacy between QS 532 nm Nd:YAG and long pulsed (LP) 532 nm Nd:YAG, but a higher risk of postoperative hyperpigmentation with the QS device. A recent study by our group comparing QS and LP alexandrite for the treatment of freckles and lentigines in 20 Chinese patients showed similar results (Fig. 10.1). There was significant improvement in pigmentation in both groups, with no difference between the groups. However, the risk of PIH was 22% in the QS group, compared with 6% in the LP group. Patients also complained of more severe pain, erythema, and edema with the QS device. These findings were further validated in a retrospective study due to be published, comparing treatment of lentigines in 40 Chinese patients with four different devices; 595 nm long pulsed dye laser (LPDL), 755 nm alexandrite laser, 532 nm QS Nd:YAG, and 532 nm LP potassium-titanyl-phosphate (KTP) laser (Fig. 10.2). The results showed that a long pulse laser and small spot size appear to reduce the risk of PIH in darker skin types (see Case study 1 at end of chapter).

LP lasers, with their longer millisecond pulse width, result in more absorption by target melanin and less absorption by competing chromophores such as oxyhemoglobin, and surrounding pigment-laden skin. This is particularly important in reducing the risk of PIH in ethnic skin. The postulated reason is that LP lasers cause melanin destruction by photothermolysis only. In contrast, QS lasers emit high-energy, nanosecond radiation, causing both photothermal and photomechanical effects. Not only is the target pigmented lesion destroyed by the short burst of intense radiation, but surrounding melanin and oxyhemoglobin are also damaged, resulting in altered activity of melanocytes, hemosiderin deposition from damaged vessels, and subsequent PIH.

Spot sizes are also an important consideration when treating darker skin types. From our retrospective study comparing four different laser devices above, we noted that when using LP alexandrite in the treatment of epidermal pigmentation in Asian skin, despite its long pulse width, significant improvement in lesional pigmentation was not found, and was associated with the highest risk of PIH (20%). We postulated that the large spot size

Figure 10.1 Representative clinical responses to the two laser treatments: (**A**) 3 months post-treatment with QS alexandrite laser; treatment parameters: 3 mm, 5 J/cm², 2 Hz. (**B**) 3 months post-treatment with LP alexandrite laser; treatment parameters: 4 mm, 13 J/cm², 2 Hz.

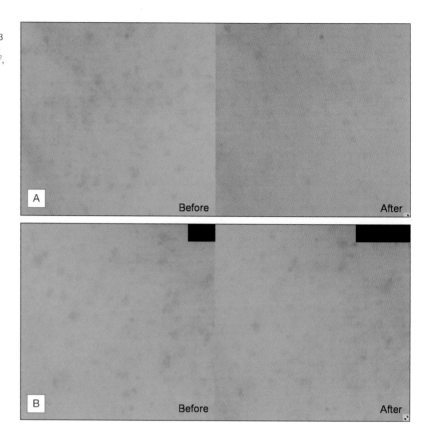

(10 mm) in the LP alexandrite laser may have led to inadvertent treatment of surrounding unaffected skin, when the lesion treated is smaller than the spot size available, and this is especially pertinent in ethnic skin where contrast between the lesional and non-lesional skin is low.

There is increasing evidence to support the use of diascopy during laser treatment to reduce the risk of PIH. This is especially true when using pigment lasers that target both oxyhemoglobin and melanin such as the LPDL. Compression of the skin surface by the flat glass window on the handpiece leads to emptying of blood vessels, reducing the risk of vascular damage, and subsequent purpura, hemosiderin deposition, and PIH. The effectiveness of such simple diascopy is supported by results from studies carried out by Kono et al, who conducted different studies using 595 nm LPDL, repeatedly demonstrating its effectiveness and safety when used with compression for the treatment of lentigines in ethnic skin, when compared with IPL and QS ruby laser. Our retrospective study also showed that 595 nm LPDL and 532 nm LP KTP, both of which utilize a compression window, have better results and less complications compared with 532 QS Nd:YAG and 755 nm LP alexandrite laser.

Intense pulsed light (IPL) sources emit a broadband of visible light (400–1200 nm) from a non-coherent filtered flashlamp and target melanin through photothermal effects. Negishi et al carried out two studies looking at photorejuvenation using IPL. Results from the first study involving 97 Asian patients showed that more than 90% reported a reduction in pigmentation after three to six treatments at intervals of 2–3 weeks (cutoff filter 550 nm, 28–32 J/cm², double pulse mode of 2.5–4.0/4.0–5.0 ms, delay time 20/40 ms). The second study used IPL with an integrated cooling system and found 80% of the 73 patients had a significant reduction in pigmentation after three to five treatments at intervals of 3–4 weeks (cutoff filter 560 nm, 23–27 J/cm², double pulse mode of 2.8–3.2/6.0 ms, delay time 20/40 ms). Kawada et al also treated lentigines and freckles in 60 patients with IPL and reported more than 50% improvement in 68% of these patients after three to five treatments at intervals of 2–3 weeks. No PIH was reported in any of these studies. A further split face study comparing QS alexandrite and IPL for freckles and lentigines in Asians found significant improvement with the QS device. However, the risk of PIH was also higher with the QS device, especially in patients with lentigines. No PIH was seen in the IPL group. These studies serve to highlight IPL, through photothermal effects, is effective and safe in the treatment of epidermal pigmentation in ethnic skin. However, multiple treatments are required. Furthermore, with a large spot size, if the contrast between the lesional and non-lesional skin is low, the therapeutic window is much narrower. Either the operator uses suboptimal energy leading to

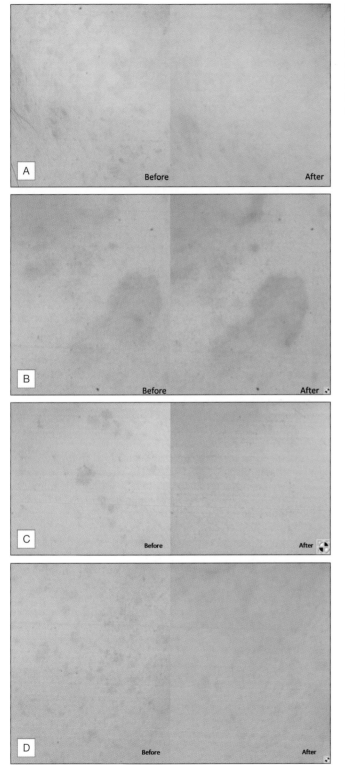

Figure 10.2 Management of freckles and lentigines with different pigment-specific lasers: (**A**) Marked improvement after two treatments with 595 nm LPDL; treatment parameters: 7 J/cm², 10 mm, 6 ms, cooling 3. (**B**) PIH post single LP alexandrite laser treatment; treatment parameters: 25 J/cm², 1.5 Hz, 3 × 10 mm, DCD 0/20/0, 3 ms. (**C**) After three treatments with LP 532 nm Nd:YAG; treatment parameters: 2 mm, 13 J/cm², 2 ms, 1 Hz. (**D**) After three treatments with LP 532nm Nd:YAG; treatment parameters: 2 mm, 13 J/cm², 2 ms, 1 Hz.

Figure 10.3 (**A**) Nevus of Ota at baseline and (**B**) after six treatments with QS 1064 nm Nd:YAG laser; treatment parameters: 12 J/cm², 10 Hz, 2 mm.

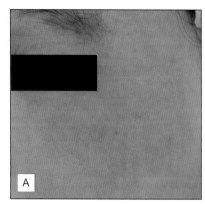
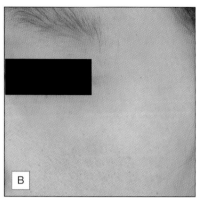

minimal effectiveness, or above threshold energy that may lead to greater risk of injury to surrounding normal skin.

Pearl 1

When the contrast between lesional and non-lesional skin is low, a small spot size allows treatment of lesion without inadvertent injury to surrounding normal skin.

Pearl 2

Long-pulsed lasers are associated with fewer complications than QS lasers, but require more treatment sessions.

A treatment algorithm for epidermal pigmentation is as follows:

1. IPL can be recommended for patients who are intolerant of any PIH risk, and are amenable to having several treatment sessions.
2. LP lasers are effective, yet require fewer treatments than IPL, and carry a low PIH risk.
3. The more aggressive approach using QS lasers only requires one to two sessions, but carries the highest risk of PIH and downtime of a week. This should be reserved for patients with time and cost constraints.

Treatment of dermal pigmentation

Dermal pigmentation such as Nevus of Ota and acquired bilateral nevus of Ota-like macules (ABNOM) or Hori's macules are much more commonly encountered in ethnic skin. Removal of unwanted tattoos and hair require the removal of dermal pigment. In such conditions, devices with longer wavelengths, and hence deeper penetration, are utilized to provide enhanced clearance.

Nevus of Ota

Nevus of Ota is an oculodermal melanocytosis affecting approximately 0.6% of the Asian population at birth or developing in their teens. Clinically, it presents as a bluish-black hyperpigmentation along the ophthalmic or maxillary branches of the trigeminal nerve. QS lasers, including QS ruby, QS alexandrite, and QS 1064 nm Nd:YAG, have all been used to achieve good therapeutic results. Watanabe and Takahashi looked at 114 nevus of Ota patients treated with QS Ruby and reported a good to excellent degree of lightening after three or more sessions. Kono et al confirmed the findings when he reviewed 101 nevus of Ota patients treated with QS Ruby and reported 56% achieving 75% improvement, and 36% achieving complete clearing. Hypopigmentation was seen in 17% of patients and hyperpigmentation in 6%. Studies comparing the use of QS alexandrite and QS 1064 nm Nd:YAG found the former better tolerated but the latter more effective after three or more treatment sessions. The longer wavelength of the QS Nd:YAG targets dermal pigment effectively with minimal epidermal damage in darker skinned individuals (**Fig. 10.3**). More recently, fractionated laser technology has been added to the currently available options. Near-complete clearance of a case of nevus of Ota after serial therapy using 1064 nm QS Nd:YAG, followed by 1550 nm non-ablative fractionated erbium-doped fiber laser treatments at 2-month intervals; and a further case achieving complete clearance with sequential same day therapy with the same devices have been reported. Treatment of nevus of Ota at a younger age requires fewer treatment sessions and is associated with fewer complications compared with older patients, and early treatment is therefore recommended (see **Case study 2**). It is important to note that the risk of recurrence is estimated to be between 0.6% and 1.2%[8], which has important implications particularly when counseling pediatric patients.

Pearl 3

Patients seeking treatment for nevus of Ota should be treated at an earlier age to reduce the risk of complications and also to reduce the number of treatment sessions required.

Hori's macules or acquired bilateral nevus of Ota-like macules

Hori's macules (ABNOM) affect 0.8% of the Asian population and presents in late adulthood as bluish brown

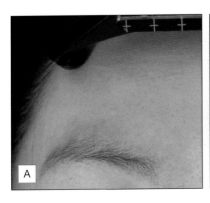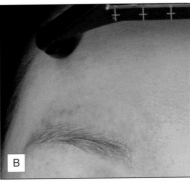

Figure 10.4 (A) Hori's macules before QS ruby treatment and **(B)** PIH post QS ruby treatment.

dermal hyperpigmentation typically affecting the bilateral malar regions, forehead and temples of middle aged women, without any mucosal involvement. QS lasers such as QS ruby, QS alexandrite and QS 1064 nm Nd:YAG have been found to be effective in the treatment of Hori's macules. More recent studies also support these results. Kagami et al reported the efficacy of QS alexandrite in 24 Japanese patients, with 45.8% reporting greater than 50% improvement. Cho et al also evaluated the use of 1064 nm QS Nd:YAG at low fluences in 15 patients, 80% of whom had greater than 50% improvement. From our experience, Hori's macules tend to be more resistant to treatment than nevus of Ota. Shorter treatment intervals every 4 weeks tend to yield better results. Combination treatment with QS 532 nm Nd:YAG, followed by QS 1064 nm Nd:YAG has also been found to be more effective than the 1064 nm wavelength alone. Transient PIH is a common adverse event, occurring in the majority of treated patients (Fig. 10.4). Permanent hypopigmentation has been reported after QS ruby treatment. In order to reduce the risk of PIH, all patients should be given pre and post-treatment bleaching agents (see Case study 3).

Pearl 4

Hori's macules require multiple treatment sessions to yield improvement. Warn patients that initial deterioration can occur, and can be treated with bleaching agents.

Tattoo removal

The removal of unwanted tattoos without scarring is now possible even in dark-skinned individuals. As different inks are present in any one tattoo, effective treatment may require the use of various wavelengths and entail multiple treatments. QS lasers are effective in removing black and blue tattoos. The longer wavelengths such as the 1064 nm QS Nd:YAG or 755 nm alexandrite laser are better suited to tattoo removal of darkly pigmented skin, as there is less absorption by epidermal melanin, and a reduced risk of subsequent dyspigmentation. Conservative initial treatment with low fluences (e.g. 1064 nm Nd:YAG, 4 mm spot size, 2.0–2.6 J/cm^2) is recommended, until the end point of whitening with no punctate bleeding is achieved.

The 694 nm QS ruby laser, although effective, can result in hyper- or permanent hypopigmentation of the skin.

Hair removal

Pigment-specific lasers with longer wavelengths, longer pulse durations and concomitant epidermal cooling have been successfully employed for hair removal in darkly pigmented skin. LP alexandrite laser, 810 nm diode, and 1064 nm Nd:YAG lasers can all be safely applied with few side effects. A recent split axilla comparison study by Wanitphakdeedecha and co-workers showed that, although both high-fluence, low-repetition 1064 nm Nd:YAG and low-fluence, high-repetition 810 nm diode laser were successful in axillary hair removal, results with the Nd:YAG were better. However, the diode laser was less painful. The use of pneumatic skin flattening has also been explored as a viable alternative to dynamic cooling device, in the reduction of pain during axillary hair removal.

Treatment of dermo-epidermal pigmentation

Common conditions where melanin is found in dermo-epidermal locations include Becker's nevus, melasma, PIH, and melanocytic nevi.

Becker's nevus

Becker's nevus commonly presents as a brown irregular patch accompanied by dark, coarse hair. It usually appears in adolescence and in males. Histologically, increased melanin is seen in the basal cells, and melanophages may be present in the papillary dermis. It is a benign condition with no reports of malignant transformation. Previously, lasers such as QS ruby and QS Nd:YAG have been shown to improve such lesions. A comparative study of the two devices showed mean clearance of at least 43% after a single treatment with either laser. Trelles et al later compared the use of Er:YAG laser and QS 1064 nm Nd:YAG in 22 patients. At 2 years' follow-up, 54% of patients ($n = 6$) achieved complete clearance after a single treatment with Er:YAG, compared with just 1 out of 11 patients reporting clearance after three treatment sessions of Nd:YAG laser. Although clinically effective, ablative laser carries a high risk of adverse effects, especially in darker skin types. QS lasers rarely achieve complete clearance, and multiple treatments are necessary. More recently, fractional resurfacing has been suggested by Glaich and colleagues as a promising new treatment modality, with two cases reporting at least 75% pigment reduction after five to six treatments with 1550 nm erbium-doped fiber laser at 4-week intervals. Long-pulsed pigment lasers have also been employed successfully to target both pigment and hair in Becker's nevus. In our experience, LP alexandrite (20–35 J/cm^2, 10 mm spot size, pulse duration 1.5 ms) gives a 50% success rate after four to eight treatments. Possible side effects include scarring and hypopigmentation. Long-pulsed pigment laser together with non-ablative fractional resurfacing with 1927 nm thulium fiber laser can lead to an optimal outcome (see Case study 4).

Melasma

Melasma is a common acquired symmetrical hypermelanosis involving sun-exposed areas commonly seen in Asian middle-aged women. Genetics, UV radiation, pregnancy, and hormonal therapies are all thought to be contributing etiological factors and it remains a challenging condition to treat. Increased pigment can be seen in either the epidermis (brownish black), or dermis (bluish gray), or both. There may also be some overlap between dermal melasma and Hori's macules (ABNOM). Wood's lamp can be useful in differentiating between the skin layers, with the pigmented epidermal layer demonstrating increased reflectance, in contrast to a lack of reflectance from the pigmented dermal layer.

In addition to sun protection and avoidance of aggravating factors such as oral contraceptives, bleaching agents remain the mainstay of treatment for melasma. Combinations of hydroquinone with topical corticosteroids and tretinoin are effective as first-line treatment. Other bleaching agents used include azelaic acid, kojic acid, arbutin, and licorice extract. Their mechanism of action includes tyrosinase inhibition, suppression of the secretory function of melanocytes, decreasing rate of transfer of melanin from melanosomes to keratinocytes, and increased epidermal turnover. Chemical peels and microdermabrasion are also useful adjuncts to topical treatments in the management of melasma in Asians.

Although laser therapy has been used to improve melasma, caution must be exercised as worsening of the disease or PIH may occur after treatment. This is likely to be due to the pathogenesis of melasma, which is believed to be due to increased activity of melanogenic enzymes, resulting in hyperactive melanocytes. Sublethal laser damage to these labile melanocytes is thought to result in an increase in melanin production and hyperpigmentation. Laser therapy should therefore be considered as second-line treatment for patients who have not improved sufficiently after 3–6 months of topical treatment.

Wang's group in Taipei examined patients with melasma treated with IPL and found a significant improvement of 39.8% in the IPL group compared with 11.6% in the control. Two patients developed transient PIH, and partial repigmentation was noted after 24 weeks, suggesting the need for repeated treatments for maintenance. They suggested the lowest fluence to achieve minimal erythema be used, which supported findings by Negishi's group. This is to avoid excessive thermal damage to labile melanocytes, which may lead to inflammation and subsequent PIH.

Pigment lasers have also been used to treat melasma. Low fluence, large spot size, multiple pass QS 1064 nm Nd:YAG, sometimes referred to as laser toning or laser facial, has become increasingly popular for the treatment of melasma. Some studies have reported it to be effective and safe, while others have highlighted important complications. Zhou et al published a recent study examining 50 patients with melasma treated with 9 weekly sessions, and reported 70% with more than 50% reduction in melasma area and severity index (MASI) values, and 10% with complete clearance. However, the recurrence rate at 3 months was 64%. Promising results were similarly reported in a prospective study by Polnikorn, after 10 weekly sessions of 1064 nm Nd:YAG in 35 refractory melasma cases. Recurrence at 6 months was seen in two cases. In addition, he noted mottled hypopigmentation occurring in three patients. Facial depigmentation is an increasingly recognized phenomenon often encountered with frequent treatments with QS 1064 nm Nd:YAG (Fig. 10. 5). Chan et al reported it in 14 Chinese patients, after a variable number of such treatments. Wattanakrai et al and Cho et al also described a similar adverse effect occurring after 1 to 2 weekly treatments with this laser for melasma, with 13.6% and 8% rate of hypopigmentation reported, respectively. With risks of recurrence and punctate hypopigmentation post-laser treatment, patients need to be adequately informed of potential complications prior to embarking on such treatments for melasma. Optimal parameters from future studies will be helpful.

Ablative resurfacing has been used with some success for the treatment of melasma. A Thai study showed promising results using variable square pulse erbium:yttrium aluminum garnet (Er:YAG) laser resurfacing in 20 patients. However, 17.6% experienced transient PIH, and recurrence was observed after the treatment was discontinued. Fractional resurfacing has been explored as a better option, with 'melanin shuttling' of underlying dermal pigment coupled with remodeling of the underlying pathologic dermis proposed as a possible mechanism. Rokhsar & Fitzpatrick piloted the use of fractional resurfacing in 10 patients, and demonstrated 60% achieved 75–100% improvement, and 30% had less than 25% improvement when treated at 1–2-week intervals for four to six treatments. A Korean study by Lee et al later showed more limited efficacy, with 60% of 25 patients reporting improvement in melasma after 4 monthly

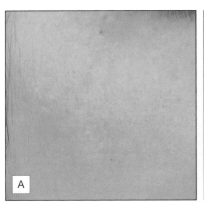

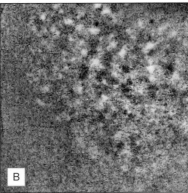

Figure 10.5 (**A**) Cross-polarized and (**B**) UV images of depigmented macules after 20 sessions of QS 1064 nm Nd:YAG laser treatment.

sessions, and improvement declining to 52.2% at 6 months; 13% of patients developed hyperpigmentation.

Due to limitations of recurrence, hyper- and hypopigmentation post-laser treatment, topical treatments remain the first line treatment for melasma, and laser treatment should only be used with caution, especially in ethnic skin.

Pearl 5

Treatment with low-fluence, large spot size QS 1064 nm laser can improve melasma. However mottled hypopigmentation can occur after repeated treatment in approximately 10% of patients.

Pearl 6

Laser and IPL should be considered as second-line treatment for patients with melasma, as there are risks of hyper and hypopigmentation, as well as recurrence.

Post-inflammatory hyperpigmentation (PIH)

PIH is characterized by an acquired increase in pigmentation secondary to an inflammatory process, and is a commonly observed response to cutaneous injury in melanin-rich Asian skin. The severity of PIH is related to the degree of inflammation and extent of disruption of the dermo-epidermal junction. Such melanogenesis is increased the darker the skin types. Histologically, excess epidermal and dermal pigmentation can be seen.

Although a benign condition, PIH can cause significant anxiety and lowered self-esteem in patients. Its initial management involves early and effective treatment of the underlying skin condition, in order to minimize any inflammation that may cause further PIH. All potential irritants such as fragrance or cosmeceuticals should be stopped. Photoprotection is imperative. Treatment modalities to accelerate the normalization of skin color include topical agents such as hydroquinone, retinoids, azelaic acid, kojic acid, glycolic and lactic acid, chemical peels, microdermabrasion, and laser treatment.

Different lasers have been used to improve PIH. Vascular lasers, such as the 595 nm LPDL, target mainly oxyhemoglobin, and can be used to treat the vascular component of the inflammatory process. When used with compression, Kono and colleagues reported that it can also be effective for pigment removal. QS lasers, such as QS Nd:YAG and QS alexandrite, have long been successfully used to treat cutaneous pigmentation. Depending on the wavelength used, epidermal and dermal pigmentation can be targeted accordingly. In recalcitrant PIH where dermal pigment may be present, 1064 nm QS Nd:YAG has been successfully used in previous reports with minimal adverse effects. More recently, our group examined the management of acne PIH in Chinese patients, and suggested the use of bleaching agents for the initial 3 months, followed by combination topical and laser therapy (LPDL and/or 1064 nm QS Nd:YAG) for recalcitrant PIH with vascular and dermal components (Fig. 10.6). Laser treatment in itself can of course be a cause of PIH in darker skin types, and strategies to reduce PIH risk include effective sun protection pre- and post-procedure, the use of long-pulsed lasers, cooling, diascopy, and small spot sizes in this group.

Melanocytic nevi

Although the gold standard for the removal of melanocytic nevi is by excision followed by histological examination, the resulting scar is often an undesired cosmetic outcome. Lasers have been used successfully to remove and lighten nevi with better cosmetic results. However, the clinician needs to be aware of the potential risk of malignant transformation, and the patient's skin type, family history, and location of lesion are important considerations. Incidence of melanoma has been reported to be between 0.2 and 2.2 per 100000 in Asians, depending on skin type. Acral regions, such as the feet, appear to be more commonly affected. Laser treatment of melanocytic nevi may therefore be considered in darker-skinned individuals with no risk factors, and lesions in a non-acral location, after an explanation of the risks involved. The combination of CO_2 and QS alexandrite laser was reported to be successful in 11 patients with congenital nevi. Further studies reported

Figure 10.6 Management of acne PIH with different treatments: (**A**) 2 months after azelaic acid 20% + Mometasone 0.1% cream + hydroquinone 4% cream. (**B**) After five treatments with QS1064 nm Nd:YAG; treatment parameters: 3.1 J/cm², 8 mm, 10 Hz.

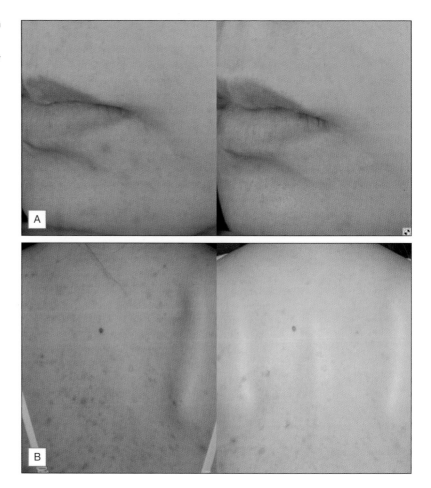

the successful use of QS ruby laser and normal mode ruby laser for acquired melanocytic nevi, particularly for flat lesions. Some compound lesions demonstrate only partial response. The use of fractional resurfacing has now been incorporated into the treatment regimen.

A typical treatment protocol is as follows: long-pulsed pigment laser (LP alexandrite 755 nm, 3 ms, 10 mm spot size, 15–25 J/cm² depending on the degree of pigmentation with slight dark gray appearance being the endpoint), to be followed immediately by QS ruby laser (4 mm spot size, 3–4 J/cm² with immediate whitening as the end point). 4–6 weeks later, the patient will be treated with non-ablative fractional resurfacing using a combination of 1550 nm and 1927 nm wavelengths (1550 nm, 4 passes, 50 mJ, treatment level 10, to be followed by 1927 nm, 4 passes, 20 mJ, treatment level 10). Such alternate treatment at 4–6 weekly intervals is performed until the nevi completely lighten (see Case study 5).

Treatment of vascular lesions

Vascular specific lasers induce vessel injury, and have been used to target vascular lesions such as port-wine stains (PWS), telangiectasia, scars as well as for non-ablative skin rejuvenation. One of the principal absorption peaks of oxyhemoglobin is at 577 nm, with a smaller peak around 700–1100 nm; 585 nm and 595 nm PDL, being close to the 577 nm peak, have shown excellent efficacy and safety in the treatment of PWS in Asians, as well as hypertrophic and keloid scars which are found more commonly in darker skin types.

Asahina et al evaluated the use of 595 nm PDL (7 mm spot size, 10 ms pulse duration, 12 J/cm²) in the treatment of PWS in skin type IV patients, and found 67% of patients achieving good or excellent results after four treatments at 8-week intervals. Hyper and hypopigmentation were seen in up to 17% and 14% respectively. Epidermal cooling and protection enhances efficacy by allowing a higher fluence to be used to achieve the desired end point of purpura with better tolerability and less side effects in darker skin types (585 nm PDL, 7 mm spot size, 1.5 ms, 7–13 J/cm², dynamic cooling device with 20 ms spray and 30 ms delay interval) (Fig. 10.7). However, complete blanching of PWS is rarely seen. It has been postulated that regeneration and revascularization of photocoagulated blood vessels due to angiogenesis occur

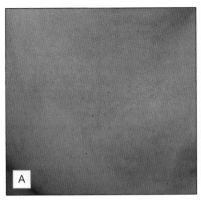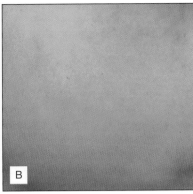

Figure 10.7 (**A**) PWS at baseline. (**B**) Marked improvement of PWS after eight LPDL treatments.

as part of the skin's normal healing process. The heterogeneity of vessels characteristic of PWS require the use of different spot sizes, fluences, pulse widths, and dynamic cooling, depending on vessel size and anatomical location. Due to a greater risk of dyspigmentation when treating lip PWS with PDL, a 1064 nm Nd:YAG is recommended. Combined 595 nm and 1064 nm laser irradiation has also been recommended for recalcitrant and hypertrophic PWS.

Long-pulsed millisecond 1064 nm Nd:YAG lasers target the lesser absoption peak of oxyhemoglobin in the infrared range and have been used in the treatment of large telangiectasia and reticular veins as they allow for deeper dermal penetration. The longer wavelength also results in minimal absorption by epidermal melanin, conferring a safe and effective treatment in patients with ethnic skin. LP 755 nm alexandrite laser has also been reported to improve vessels after a single treatment, but PIH is seen in 30% of patients, possibly due to hemosiderin deposition and/or excessive cooling.

Facial telangiectasia is a common dermatological complaint and may be associated with rosacea, photodamage, prolonged topical corticosteroid use, liver disease, radiodermatitis, and connective tissue disease. PDL is presently regarded as the treatment of choice, due to its excellent efficacy and safety profile. However, purpura and/or PIH can occur at the treated site and is generally unacceptable to most patients, and hence studies comparing the efficacy of purpuric and subpurpuric PDL treatment for facial telangiectasia. In a split face study by Alam and colleagues, purpuric settings achieved a greater reduction in telangiectasia density in 82% of patients (7 mm spot size, 10 ms pulse duration, fluence 8.5 to 10 J/cm², DCD 30 ms spray and 20 ms delay interval). Another study by Jasim and co-workers showed subpurpuric treatment with PDL (7 mm spot size, pulse duration 6 ms, fluence 7 to 9 J/cm²) resulted in 75% of patients achieving greater than 25% improvement after a single treatment. This is generally preferred due to minimal downtime, although the lack of a visible end point may lead to subtherapeutic treatment and the need for more treatments to achieve the desired outcome. Further studies have suggested the use

of dual-wavelength laser treatments with sequential subpurpuric delivery of 595 nm and 1064 nm radiation demonstrating better results when compared with single wavelength treatment after a single treatment session.

The use of PDL has additionally been proven to be effective in the treatment of hypertrophic scars and keloids, which are more common in darker-skinned patients. Improvements in skin texture, bulk, and scar texture have been reported. In patients with highly melanized skin, lower fluences are used to minimize PIH. Relatively low energy (10 mm spot size, 0.45–1.5 ms, 4.5–5.0 J/cm²) at 2-month intervals are utilized when using PDL to treat hypertrophic scars in ethnic skin, and in thin skinned areas such as the chest and neck. Epidermal skin cooling can also help to reduce the risk of dyspigmentation.

Ablative, non-ablative, and fractional skin resurfacing

Ablative resurfacing with carbon dioxide (CO₂) and Er:YAG lasers has long been the gold standard. These target water as a chromophore, leading to epidermal and dermal vaporization and ablation of 100–200 μm in depth. Although clinically effective in improving rhytides, atrophic scarring and dyschromia, there is significant associated downtime and potential side effects, including persistent erythema, hyper- and hypopigmentation, infection, and even scarring, especially in dark skin.

Patients with darker skin are seeking alternative skin resurfacing treatments with lower risk profiles. Non-ablative lasers that deliver laser, light-based or radiofrequency energy to the skin have been the focus of the shift in recent years, and these include PDL, IPL, Nd:YAG, diode, and Er:glass lasers. Modest improvement in skin texture, scars, and rhytides is typically produced after a series of monthly treatments using these devices. There is little downtime associated and adverse effects such as PIH and scarring are much less when compared with ablative devices.

Radiofrequency has been used successfully for non-invasive skin rejuvenation. The radiofrequency device

Figure 10.8 (**A**) Baseline and (**B**) 5 months after monopolar radiofrequency for skin tightening.

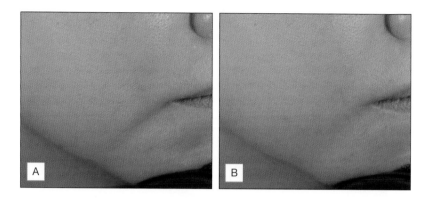

Figure 10.9 (**A**) Baseline and (**B**) 3 months after focused ultrasound treatment; treatment parameter: 1.2 J.

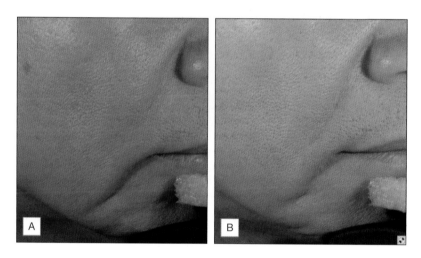

delivers an electric current that nonselectively generates heat by the tissue's natural resistance to the flow of ions. Epidermal cooling from the cooling tip protects against melanin disruption, and radiofrequency can be safely applied to any skin type. Such delivery of energy deep into 2–4 mm of the dermis induces subtle collagen damage and subsequent healing and remodeling, resulting in immediate skin tightening, and further improvement after several months. Monopolar radiofrequency is considered the gold standard in non-invasive skin tightening but can be limited by pain issues (Fig. 10.8). Patient feedback on heat sensation is thought to be a valid and preferred method for optimal energy selection. Multiple passes at moderate energy settings have yielded good and consistent results. Newer models have incorporated a vibrating handpiece, in order to reduce the sensation of pain, in accordance with the gate theory.

Focused ultrasound is another new technology that translates ultrasound into thermal energy; in addition, it allows imaging of the tissue before application of the focused ultrasound directly to the target area. A preliminary study on 49 Chinese patients has shown early promising results with significant improvement to the lower face and a good safety profile with only transient bruising, erythema, edema, and PIH described (Fig. 10.9).

The development of fractional photothermolysis has revolutionized skin rejuvenation and resurfacing, attempting to achieve comparable clinical results to ablative lasers, but with a safety profile more similar to non-ablative technologies. The 1550 nm erbium-doped fiber non-ablative laser is the first fractional laser approved for clinical use. By creating an array of microscopic treatment zones (MTZs) with controlled width, depth, and density, a fixed percentage of the skin is thermally coagulated in each treatment session, leaving an intact stratum corneum. Healthy tissue surrounding these MTZs allow for rapid healing and re-epithelialization within 1 day. This technology has proven to be effective in improving photoaging, dyschromia, rhytides, atrophic scarring, and poikiloderma. Non-ablative fractional resurfacing (NA FR) used for acne scarring in Asian skin carries a high risk of PIH. Studies have indicated that treatment density, rather than energy, is a stronger determining factor in the development of PIH. Further studies by Chan and colleagues have confirmed that by reducing the number of passes and the total treatment density (four rather than eight passes), but increasing the treatment sessions from three to six to compensate for the reduced passes, clinical efficacy remains statistically improved whilst reducing the PIH risk in Asians from 18.2% to 6% (Fig. 10.10).

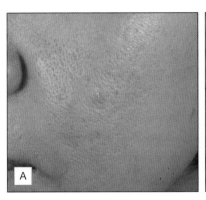
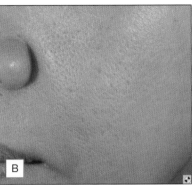

Figure 10.10 (**A**) Acne scarring at baseline and (**B**) 1 month after 8 NA FR treatments with four passes during each treatment; treatment parameters: pulse energy 60 mJ, total energy 3.05 kJ, total density 125 MTZ/cm^2.

Pearl 7

In non-ablative fractional resurfacing, reducing the treatment density and increasing the number of treatment sessions can reduce the PIH risk in ethnic skin.

More recently, ablative fractional resurfacing (AFR) has been investigated for photorejuvenation and acne scarring in Asian skin. Preliminary studies using a fractional CO_2 ablative device on nine Chinese patients found improvement in skin texture, skin laxity, wrinkles, enlarged pores, and acne scars, with 55.5% and 11.1% PIH risk at 1 and 6 months, respectively.

Case studies

CASE STUDY 1
Freckles and lentigo

A 55-year-old female who enjoys outdoor activities and sunbathing presents with troubling pigmentation on her face (Fig. 10.11A–D), which has been increasing in numbers in recent years. She does not use sunscreens and continues to play golf on a regular basis. She has a busy job that requires her to meet with clients on a daily basis and requests a treatment with little downtime.

Examination reveals Type III skin with multiple freckles on both cheeks and a large lentigo over her left zygoma. Different pigment laser options were discussed with the patient. The importance of sun avoidance 2 weeks before and after treatment was emphasized.

As she wants an effective treatment with a low risk of PIH, the long-pulsed KTP 532 nm laser (10.5–11 J/cm^2, 3 mm spot size, pulse duration 2 ms) was used to target her unwanted epidermal pigmentation. She showed good improvement after two treatment sessions. She was given the appropriate sun protection advice, and prescribed daily sunscreen. Further treatment sessions can be considered if further lightening of her pigmentation is required.

CASE STUDY 2
Nevus of Ota

A 23-year-old Chinese male presents with a bluish-gray patch over his left forehead, temple, malar area, and periorbital skin (Fig. 10.12A,B). It has been present since infancy and has gradually enlarged and darkened in color over the years. It has, however, been stable since he reached adulthood and he is keen to have it treated.

Examination showed a nevus of Ota over the distribution of the left ophthalmic branch of the trigeminal nerve. It is unilateral and does not involve the sclera. His diagnosis and treatment options were discussed and it was explained that multiple treatments with longer wavelength pigment lasers would be helpful for his dermal melanosis. The risks of hyper- and hypopigmentation post-laser were also discussed.

The patient gave informed consent for treatment to be carried out and underwent seven treatments with QS Nd:YAG 1064 nm laser (10–12 J/cm^2, 2 mm spot size) at 4–6 weeks' interval, followed by four sessions of QS ruby (3.1–3.6 J/cm^2, 5 mm spot size) also at 4–6 weeks' interval. He achieved an excellent result and is highly satisfied with his treatment.

CASE STUDY 3
Hori's macules

A 28-year-old Chinese female presents with speckled dark pigmentation over her malar cheeks (Fig. 10.13A,B). She noticed this only in the last 2 years and worries that it may darken further. She does not use regular sunscreen.

Examination confirmed the presence of Hori's macules on both malar cheeks. There was no mucosal involvement. A discussion with the patient explored treatment options and it was explained that several laser treatments are required for this resistant dermal condition. The risk of hyperpigmentation after initial laser treatment before subsequent lightening after further treatment was highlighted. She consented and underwent three sessions of QS ruby laser (3.4 J/cm^2, long tip 5 mm) and a further session with QS alexandrite 755 nm laser (8.5 J/cm^2, 3 mm). Bleaching topical agents were used in between treatments. She achieved and maintained significant lightening 3 months after her last treatment.

Figure 10.11 Improvement in epidermal pigmentation after treatment with the long-pulsed 532 nm laser.

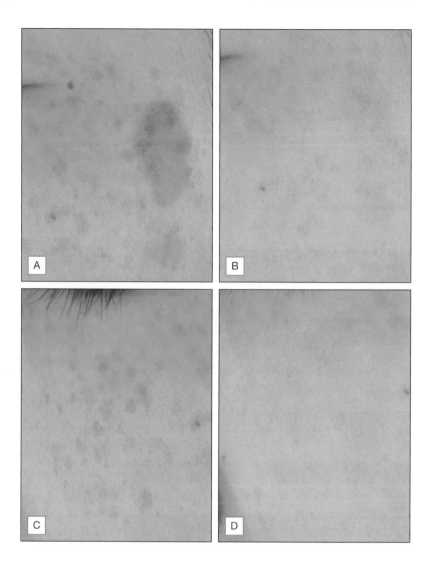

Figure 10.12 Marked improvement of nevus of ota after combination treatment with Q-switched 1064 nm laser and Q-switched Ruby.

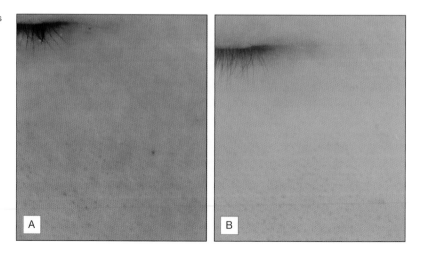

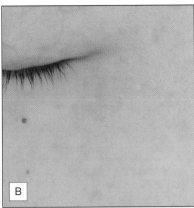

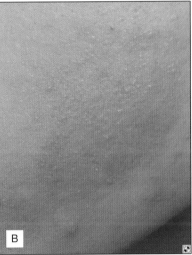

Figure 10.13 Lightening of Hori's macules after treatment with Q-switched ruby laser and Q-switched Alexandrite 755 nm laser.

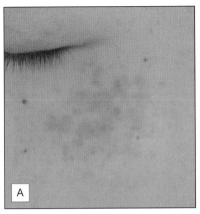

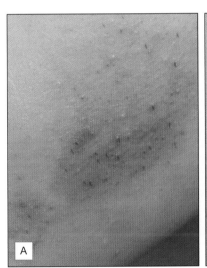

Figure 10.14 Improvement in Becker's nevus after treatment with long-pulsed Alexandrite laser and non-ablative fractional resurfacing with 1927 nm Thulium fiber laser.

CASE STUDY 4
Becker's nevus

A 27-year-old male developed a hairy, pigmented area on his left jaw during his teens and presented requesting its removal (Fig. 10.14A,B). It has not changed in size or darkened in recent years, but he is highly troubled by its cosmetic appearance.

Examination showed a large irregular brown patch with several dark hairs over his left jaw. A Becker's nevus was diagnosed and the patient was treated with LP alexandrite laser (20–30 J/cm^2, 10 mm spot size, pulse duration 1.5 ms). He underwent four treatments at 4–6-week intervals. He also underwent two sessions of non-ablative fractional resurfacing with a 1927 nm thulium fiber laser (treatment level 11, eight passes) to achieve further improvement. A faint brown patch remains and the patient is satisfied with the improvement in appearance.

CASE STUDY 5
Melanocytic nevi

A 34-year-old Chinese male requested that two moles on his right cheek be removed (Fig. 10.15A,B). He has no family history of any skin malignancies and his moles have not changed for several years. Examination showed a dark-brown junctional nevus and another brown compound nevus on his cheek. During the consultation, the need for multiple treatments and risk of PIH was discussed. It was also explained that there may not be complete clearance and recurrence may occur.

The patient underwent treatment with three sessions of LP alexandrite (20 J/cm^2, 3 × 10 mm spot size, 3 ms) followed by three sessions of QS ruby (3.2–3.4 J/cm^2, 4 mm spot size) at 4–6-weekly intervals until the nevi have sufficiently lightened.

Figure 10.15 Successful lightening of melanocytic nevi with long-pulsed Alexandrite and Q-switched Ruby laser.

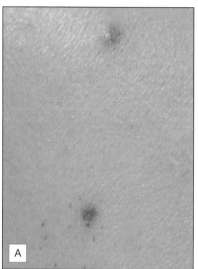
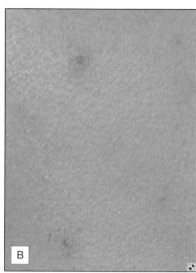

Conclusion

With the rapid evolution of demographics globally, increasing numbers of patients with ethnic skin will present to dermatologists seeking laser treatment for cosmetic enhancement. Understanding and establishing treatment protocols with appropriate parameters for all skin types is essential in the running of a successful practice.

Further reading

Alam M, Dover JS, Arndt KA 2003 Treatment of facial telangiectasia with variable-pulse high-fluence pulsed-dye laser: comparison of efficacy with fluences immediately above and below the purpura threshold. Dermatologic Surgery 29:681-685

Asahina A, Watanabe T, Kishi A, et al 2006 Evaluation of the treatment of port-wine stains with the 595 nm long pulsed dye laser: a large prospective study in adult Japanese patients. Journal of the American Academy of Dermatology 54:487-493

Chan HH, Fung WKK, Ying SY, et al 2000 An in vivo trial comparing the use of different types of 532 nm Nd:YAG lasers in the treatment of facial lentigines in Oriental patients. Dermatologic Surgery 26(8):743-749

Chan NP, Ho SG, Yeung CK, et al 2010 The use of non-ablative fractional resurfacing in Asian acne scar patients. Lasers in Surgery and Medicine 42(10):710-715

Chan NPY, Ho SGY, Shek SYN, et al 2010 A case series of facial depigmentation associated with low fluence Q-switched 1064 nm Nd:YAG laser for skin rejuvenation and melasma. Lasers in Surgery and Medicine 42(8):712-719

Cho SB, Park SJ, Kim MJ, et al 2009 Treatment of acquired bilateral nevus of Ota-like macules (Hori's nevus) using 1064 nm Q-switched Nd:YAG with low fluence. International Journal of Dermatology 48:1308-1312

Dufresne RG, Phillips KA, Vittorio CC, et al 2001 A screening questionnaire for body dysmorphic disorder in a cosmetic surgery practice. Dermatologic Surgery 27:457-462

Glaich AS, Goldberg LH, Dai T, et al 2007 Fractional resurfacing: a new therapeutic modality for Becker's nevus. Archives of Dermatology 143:1488-1490

Ho SG, Yeung CK, Chan NP, et al 2011 A retrospective analysis of the management of acne post-inflammatory hyperpigmentation using topical treatment, laser treatment, or combination topical and laser treatments in oriental patients. Lasers in Surgery and Medicine 43(1):1-7

Ho SGY, Yeung CK, Chan NPY, et al 2011 A comparison of Q-switched and long-pulsed alexandrite laser for the treatment of freckles and lentigines in oriental patients. Lasers in Surgery and Medicine 43(2):108-113

Jasim ZF, Woo WK, Handley JM 2004 Long-pulsed (6-ms) pulsed dye laser treatment of rosacea-associated telangiectasia using subpurpuric clinical threshold. Dermatologic Surgery 30:37-40

Kagami S, Asahina A, Watanabe R, et al 2007 Treatment of 153 Japanese patients with Q-switched alexandrite laser. Lasers in Medical Science 22:159-163

Kawada A, Shiraishi H, Asai M, et al 2002 Clinical improvement of solar lentigines and ephelides with an intense pulsed light source. Dermatol Surg 28:504-508

Kono T, Chan HH, Groff WF, et al 2007 Long-pulse pulsed dye laser delivered with compression for treatment of facial lentigines. Dermatologic Surgery 33:945-950

Kono T, Nozaki M, Chan HH, et al 2001 A retrospective study looking at the long-term complications of Q-switched ruby laser in the treatment of nevus of Ota. Lasers in Surgery and Medicine 29:156-159

Lee HS, Won CH, Lee DH, et al 2009 Treatment of melasma in Asian skin using a fractional 1550 nm laser: an open clinical study. Dermatologic Surgery 35:1499-1504

Negishi K, Kushikata N, Tezuka Y, et al 2004 Study of the incidence and nature of 'very subtle epidermal melasma' in relation to intense pulsed light treatment. Dermatologic Surgery 30:881-886

Negishi K, Tezuka Y, Kushikata N, et al 2001 Photorejuvenation for Asian skin by intense pulse light. Dermatologic Surgery 27:627-632

Negishi K, Wakamatsu S, Kushikata N, et al 2002 Full-face photorejuvenation of photodamaged skin by intense pulsed light with integrated contact cooling: initial experiences in Asian patients. Lasers in Surgery and Medicine 30:298-305

Polnikorn N 2010 Treatment of refractory melasma with the MedLite C6 Q-switched Nd:YAG laser and alpha arbutin: a prospective study. Cosmetic Laser Therapy 12:126-131

Rokhsar CK, Fitzpatrick RE 2005 The treatment of melasma with fractional photothermolysis: a pilot study. Dermatologic Surgery 31:1645-1650

Trelles MA, Allones I, Moreno-Arias GA, et al 2005 Becker's naevus: a comparative study between erbium:YAG and Q-switched neodymium:YAG; clinical and histopathological findings. British Journal of Dermatology 152:308-313

Wang CC, Hui CY, Sue YM, et al 2004 Intense pulsed light for the treatment of refractory melasma in Asian patients. Dermatologic Surgery 30:1196-1200

Wanitphakdeedecha R, Thanomkitti K, Sethabutra P, et al 2011 A split axilla comparison study of axillary hair removal with low fluence high repetition rate 810 nm diode laser vs. high fluence low repetition rate 1064 nm Nd:YAG laser. Journal of the European Academy of Dermatology and Venereology Sep 19 (Epub ahead of print)

Watanabe S, Takahashi H 1994 Treatment of nevus of Ota with the Q-switched ruby laser. New England Journal of Medicine 331:1745-1750

Zhou X, Gold MH, Lu Z, et al 2011 Efficacy and safety of Q-switched 1064 nm neodymium-doped yttrium aluminium garnet laser treatment of melasma. Dermatologic Surgery 37(7):962-970

11

Complications and legal considerations of laser and light treatments

David J. Goldberg, Jeremy Man

Summary and Key Features

- Complications
- Lasers
- Light sources
- Scars
- Pigmentary changes
- Negligence
- Standard of care
- Duty
- Breach of duty
- Causation
- Damages
- Medical malpractice
- Expert witness

Introduction

Laser and light therapy is a constantly evolving and improving area within the medical field. Although lasers were initially developed with medical purposes in mind, the gradual shift has been towards cosmetics. The variety of lasers and light treatments available can treat such things as wrinkles, scars, vascular lesions, unwanted hair, pigmentary disturbances, tattoos and medical conditions such as psoriasis, vitiligo, and acne. There are a few general points in terms of laser and light therapy that will be discussed, after which more specific points will be made.

Complications are adverse events or responses to a therapy or procedure. Many complications that can arise are not laser specific; however, there are some complications that are more likely to arise with certain laser and light procedures. A more general discussion leading to a more focused discussion on complications within certain subsets of lasers will follow.

Pearl 1

Complications are adverse events or responses to a therapy or procedure.

General considerations

It is beyond the scope of this chapter to discuss the specifics in setting up a laser unit. However, there are a number of medical–legal issues that can arise if laser treatments are done in unaccredited facilities, by untrained staff, or without the proper safety equipment.

Accreditation is a voluntary process by which a facility is able to measure itself against nationally recognized standards. There are several organizations through which a facility can accredit itself. The American Osteopathic Association (AOA), the Joint Commission on Accreditation of Health Care Organizations (JCAHO) and the Accreditation Association for Ambulatory Health Care (AAAHC) all accredit organizations and facilities.

Displaying certificates of accreditation serves as a reassurance to patients, the public, and to other healthcare professionals that a facility has met an independent standard of quality.

The geographic location of where treatments are done will determine the regulations of who can utilize a laser or light device. Each regulatory board has different rules. In some jurisdictions, only a physician may legally operate a laser or light device. Other jurusdictions require a certain amount of training and certification. Some require that a physician has evaluated the patient before the procedure is performed. It is up to the individuals involved to find out the established rules of their jurisdiction.

Eye protection within the workplace is mandated depending on location. In the US, guidance for protective eyewear is outlined by the American National Standards Institute (ANSI) Z136 series. This is published and constructed by the Laser Institute of America (LIA). In Europe, eye protection guidelines are outlined in the EN 207. Further suggestions include warning signs on the door to warn anyone entering the operating room.

Complications

The many mechanisms of action of various laser and light sources lead to the potential for many different complications. Some lead to more frequent and/or more serious complications. However, many laser and light devices work by the principles of selective photothermolysis, and thus these complications can be discussed together.

General complications

The most common complications of laser treatment are: burning, prolonged erythema, hypo- or hyperpigmentation, reactivation of herpes simplex virus, and acneiform eruption.

Burning can be a common complication of a variety of lasers. Burning can occur with the use of vascular, hair removal, and non-ablative rejuvenation lasers as well as intense pulsed light (IPL) devices. When a burn occurs, it is usually due to one of three possible causes: too high a fluence, too short a pulse duration, or insufficient epidermal cooling. Most lasers have initial recommended settings, which are fairly safe parameters with appropriate technique and adequate epidermal cooling. Depending on the severity of the burn, there is usually little that is required in terms of treatment. With only a slight burn, there may be prolonged erythema. With a more severe burn, however, blistering and scarring may develop. Occurrences of more severe hypertrophic scarring have been minimized with the advent of newer technology and the disuse of more scar-prone lasers such as the continuous wave argon laser.

Prolonged erythema can be defined in a number of ways. Erythema is an expected result with the use of most lasers. The duration of erythema is often only 24–72 hours. Prolonged erythema has been reported with all laser and light devices. In general, no treatment is required except reassurance. Non-ablative lasers generally have a shorter duration of erythema, whereas ablative resurfacing lasers have a higher rate of persistent erythema, which can last from weeks to several months.

Hyperpigmentation (Fig. 11.1) is a very common complication and possibly the most common in darker skin types (see the study by Sriprachya-anunt and colleagues).

It has been described with the use of almost every laser and light device in darker skin types. In one study by Moreno-Arias and co-workers, it was observed in 16% of patients undergoing IPL treatment. Goh reported that it can be as high as 45% in patients with skin types IV–VI. Wareham et al reported that the pulse dye laser can cause hyperpigmentation, especially on the lower legs and where there is inadequate post-treatment sun protection and sun avoidance. Hyperpigmentation was also seen by Chowdhury and colleagues with the KTP laser. With the ablative CO_2 laser, post-inflammatory hyperpigmentation (PIH) is common and was reported by Badawi et al to occur in 20–30% of Fitzpatrick III and 100% of Fitzpatrick IV patients. Mahmoud et al found the Er:YAG laser to have a PIH rate of 50% in patients with skin type IV–V (Fig. 11.2). Even non-ablative fractional lasers can cause problems with PIH; in a 2010 study by Chan et al there was an 18.2% rate in 47 patients treated. Although rarer, PIH has also been reported (e.g. by Choudhary et al and Kuperman-Beade et al) to occur with the use of Q-switched lasers. In darker skin types, it can be fairly common; it was reported by Lapidoth & Aharonowitz to occur in up to 44% of darker-skinned patients. As noted above, vascular lasers were also found by Clark et al to result in PIH, albeit more rarely.

Hypopigmentation is a less common complication and is most commonly seen with the use of Q-switched lasers for tattoo removal as well as vascular lasers for port-wine stains. Hypopigmentation from Q-switched lasers may be transient, but it can also be permanent. Depigmentation was also reported (by Fitzpatrick & Goldman) to occur with Q-switched lasers. In the treatment of port-wine stains, the pulse dye laser has incidence rates of 2–31% of hypopigmentation. Longer pulse durations with the pulse dye laser seem to lessen the possibility of this complication. The ablative lasers have all been found to cause hypopigmentation (e.g. studies by Trelles and by Ward & Baker). Permanent hypopigmentation has also been described with the use of the CO_2 laser and, in a recent 10-year follow-up study by Prado and colleagues, 8.7% of patients had problems with permanent hypopigmentation.

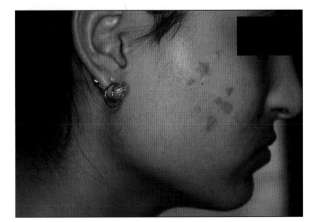

Figure 11.1 Post-inflammatory hyperpigmentation following treatment with the Q-switched Nd:YAG laser.

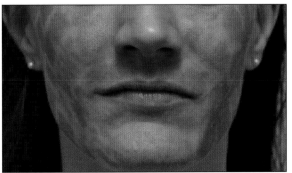

Figure 11.2 Post-inflammatory hyperpigmentation following treatment with the erbium:YAG laser.

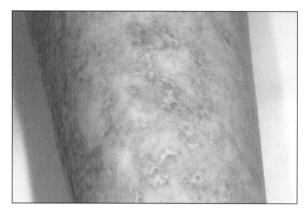

Figure 11.3 Hypopigmentation and scarring following treatment with the pulsed dye laser.

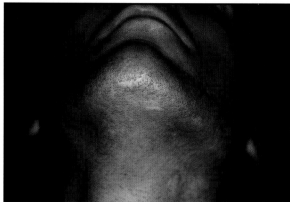

Figure 11.5 Scarring following laser hair removal.

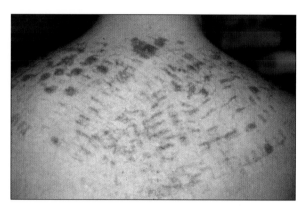

Figure 11.4 Scarring following treatment with the carbon dioxide laser.

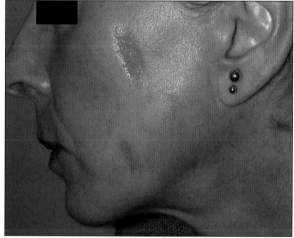

Figure 11.6 Scarring following treatment with an intense pulsed light.

Reactivation of herpes simplex virus (HSV) is a possible complication for which prophylactic antivirals are often given, especially with resurfacing lasers. However, in a recent retrospective study by Trelles of patients not given antiviral prophylaxis, less than 1% of 600 patients developed reactivation of HSV with the use of a resurfacing laser. In another retrospective study by Campbell & Goldman, only 1.1% of 373 patients developed herpes reactivation with fractionated CO_2 laser resurfacing. Despite a low incidence rate, the potential for scarring with disseminated HSV infection can make this a serious complication.

Acneiform eruptions can occur with any laser and light device and may be due to either procedure or after care. Reported rates depend on the treatment, but in the three studies by Campbell & Goldman, Nanni & Alster, and Neaman et al they ranged from 3 to 15% of patients with resurfacing lasers. This is a relatively benign complication with self-resolution expected.

Scarring has been reported with almost every cutaneous laser and light source (Figs 11.3–11.6). The actual incidence is fairly small, yet overaggressive treatment with any laser or light device can cause it. Hypertrophic scarring is most common with the older continuous wave lasers, most of which are no longer commonly used in office practice.

Specific laser complications

The complications covered above are common to almost all laser and light devices. However, there are some specific complications or considerations of various subsets of lasers.

Q-switched lasers

In the study by Kuperman-Beade and co-workers, the most common adverse effects of the Q-switched lasers included hypo- and hyperpigmentation, textural change, and scarring after treatment (see Fig. 11.1). Melanin is the main competing chromophore and transient hypopigmentation as well as permanent depigmentation with the Q-switched ruby laser can be seen (see the study above and those by Bernstein and Choudhary et al). Grevelink et al found that the Q-switched Nd:YAG laser with its longer wavelength has less chance of hypopigmentation than the Q-switched ruby laser. In darker-skinned individuals, if a Q-switched laser other than the Nd:YAG laser is used then decreasing the fluence may help prevent hypopigmentation, according to Kuperman-Beade et al.

Hyperpigmentation is less common with the Q-switched lasers than hypopigmentation; however, Choudhary et al found that bleaching agents may help prevent this in the treatment of darker-skinned individuals, and that the use of longer wavelength lasers may also minimize hyperpigmentation. Textural change is rarer and can be seen with an incidence of up to 12% with the alexandrite laser, as reported in the study by Fitzpatrick & Goldman.

A rarer but reported side effect is an allergic reaction post-treatment. In studies by Kuperman-Beade et al, England et al, and Ashinoff et al, this was mostly seen with red cinnabar pigment and can present as a nodular scaly pruritic eruption or as an immediate urticarial eruption. Ashinoff et al reported that this may be secondary to extracellular dispersal of tattoo pigment.

Paradoxical tattoo pigment darkening is a well-recognized possible complication when treating red, pink, skin tone, and white dyes. Kuperman-Beade et al found that it can rarely also happen with blue, green, and yellow dyes. The reduction of ferric and titanium dioxide are thought to be the causative factor in this darkening. This darkening is often resistant to further treatment by Q-switched lasers. Further, Arndt et al found that Q-switched laser treatment in a patient with any history of gold salt ingestion will produce a permanent dark blue dyspigmentation know as chrysiasis. Chrysiasis can be challenging to treat. Addtionally, transient immune reactions were seen by Izikson et al with laser treatment.

A rare but very serious complication is compartment syndrome. This was reported by Kuperman-Beade et al and by Rheingold et al in the circumferential treatment of the forearm with a Q-switched Nd:YAG laser.

Fractionated non-ablative lasers

The fractionated non-ablative lasers are well tolerated in most patients and have few complications. Hardaway and co-workers found that usually only mild, transient pain, erythema, and edema are seen. Studies by Chan et al, Laubach et al, and Tanzi et al concluded that dyschromia is fairly uncommon compared with standard ablative lasers. To halve the risk of PIH, Chan and colleagues recommended that the MTZ density be decreased by half and more treatments are given. Blistering, acneiform eruptions, milia, reactivation of HSV infections, and scarring are rare complications.

Ablative lasers

The ablative lasers have come a long way in terms of safety. From continuous wave to pattern scanner to fractionated technology, technology has continuously been updated to improve safety while retaining efficacy.

Continuous wave CO_2 lasers had a high incidence of scarring and hypertrophic scarring along with pigmentary disturbances.

For the most part, fractionated technology is being used in combination with ablative lasers to improve safety. However, even with fractionation, hypertrophic scarring of the neck has been reported (e.g. by Avram et al with fractionated CO_2 laser resurfacing).

Long-term hypopigmentation in the use of CO_2 laser resurfacing was reported by Ward & Baker. It seems to be more common in fair-skinned individuals There is some evidence (by Grimes et al) that hypopigmentation is a result of suppressed melanogenesis rather than true destruction of melanocytes, and treatment with the excimer laser was shown by Raulin to repigment hypopigmented areas. Transient ectropion has additionally been reported by Neaman et al to occur very rarely as a potential complication. Milia also occurred in Nanni & Alster's study in up to 10% of patients after resurfacing; this can easily be treated with standard extraction.

Infections are fairly uncommon, but can be bacterial, viral and/or fungal, as found in the study by Alam et al. Dissemination of the wart virus with transient eruption and subsequent self-resolution has been described by Torezan and colleagues. Abscess formation with *Mycobacterium fortuitum* 1 month after CO_2 laser resurfacing was also reported by Rao and co-workers.

Vascular lasers

The vascular lasers have become safer over time. The advent of pulsed rather than continuous lasers, better cooling technology, and the understanding of selective photothermolysis have advanced the safety profile tremendously. However, there are still a few complications commonly seen. Purpura is expected with the use of the pulse dye laser with short pulse durations and high fluences. Iyer & Fitzpatrick reported that lower fluences with multiple passes or cautious pulse stacking can be performed to achieve similar results without purpura. Long pulse durations can also eliminate post-treatment purpura. Rarely, there can be textural change, with an incidence of less than 1% in the treatment of port-wine stains in the studies by Kono et al and Levine & Geronemus (see **Fig. 11.3**). The latter also found that PIH can be common if there is sunlight exposure post-treatment, so sun avoidance or protection needs to be utilized. Older vascular lasers had a much higher incidence of complications, with the argon laser notorious for causing atrophic hypopigmented scars. Olbricht and colleagues found another notable complication with the argon laser was hypertrophic scarring and prolonged wound healing.

IPL-specific complications

IPL treatment is very well tolerated in general, but it has a higher learning curve with an increased number of variables. These variables include filters, pulse duration, fluence, the ability to double or triple pulse, and a variety of indications. Crusting and blistering occur in approximately 2–16% of patients; further, persistent local heat sensation lasting longer than 24 hours occur in 2% of patients. A rare complication of IPL treatment seen by Vlachos & Kontoes was the development of terminal hairs within a treated port-wine stain. Scarring has been only rarely reported (see the studies by Ho et al and Raulin et al and **Fig. 11.6**). Treatment of tanned patients can produce obvious hypopigmentation. Paradoxical hair growth has been reported (by Babilas et al, and Moreno-Arias et al), along with transient hypopigmentation and post-inflammatory hyperpigmentation especially in patients with darker skin and Mediterranean or middle-eastern background. Leukotrichia was also found to develop, along with temporary color change from black to yellow color, in studies by Radmanesh et al.

Legal aspects

Regardless of training, quality of equipment, and rigidity in patient selection, it is almost inevitable that, over a lifetime, certain complications will occur in the hands of any healthcare practitioner. In most cases, these will not result in legal action. However, if legal action is taken, then the most common interaction between a healthcare operator and healthcare law is in the realm of negligence.

Four elements must be present for there to be cause of action in negligence: duty, breach of duty, causation, and damages. A suing plaintiff must show the presence of all four elements to be successful in his or her claim.

Pearl 3

Negligence requires proof of duty, breach of duty, causation and damages.

The duty of a physician performing energy-based laser or light treatments is to perform that procedure in accordance with the 'standard of care'. Although the elements of a cause of action in negligence are derived from formal legal textbooks, the standard of care is not necessarily derived from a textbook. It is also not articulated by any judge. The standard of care is defined by some as whatever an expert witness says it is and what a jury will believe. In a case against a physician performing laser/light source treatments, the specialist must have the knowledge and skill ordinarily possessed by a specialist in that field, and have used the care and skill ordinarily possessed by a specialist in that field in the same or similar locality under similar circumstances. A dermatologist, physician extender, or for that matter an internist performing these procedures will all be held to an equal standard. A failure to fulfill such a duty may lead to loss of a lawsuit by that individual. If the jury accepts the suggestion that the provider mismanaged the case and that the negligence led to damage of the patient, then liability will ensue.

Conversely, if the jury believes an expert who testifies for a defendent doctor, then the standard of care in that particular case has been met. In this view, the standard of care is a pragmatic concept, decided case by case and based on the testimony of an expert physician. The sued physician is expected to perform the procedure in a manner of a reasonable physician. He or she need not be the best in his/her field, but need only perform the procedure in a manner that is considered by an objective standard as reasonable.

It is important to note that where there are two or more recognized laser methods of treating the same condition, a physician does not fall below the standard of care by using any of the acceptable methods even if one method turns out to be less effective than another method. Finally, in many jurisdictions, an unfavorable result due to an 'error in judgment' by a physician is not in and of itself a violation of the standard of care if the physician acted appropriately prior to exercising his/her professional judgment.

Pearl 4

There may be more than one accepted laser approach. Choosing one, and not the other, is not a breach of duty.

Evidence of the standard of care in a specific malpractice case includes laws, regulations, and guidelines for practice, which represent a consensus among professionals on a topic involving diagnosis or treatment, and the medical literature including peer-reviewed articles and authoritative texts. In addition, the view of an expert is crucial. Although the standard of care may vary from state to state, it is typically defined as a national standard by the profession at large.

Most commonly, for litigation purposes, expert witnesses articulate the standard of care. The basis of the expert witness and the origin of the standard of care, is grounded in the following:

1. The witness' personal practice and/or
2. The practice of others that he has observed in his experience; and/or
3. Medical literature in recognized publications; and/or
4. Statutes and/or legislative rules; and/or
5. Courses where the subject is discussed and taught in a well-defined manner.

Pearl 5

Expert witnesses articulate the standard of care.

The standard of care is the way in which the majority of the physicians in a similar medical community would practice. It is the method by which other laser physicians deal with their daily performance of cosmetic dermatology. If, in fact, the expert does not practice like the majority of other physicians, then the expert will have a difficult time explaining why the majority of the medical community does not practice according to his/her ways.

Pearl 6

A complication is not proof of negligence.

Complications following laser- and light-based treatments can occur. They are not necessarily acts of negligence. If the treating provider acts in accordance with the standard of care, it is unlikely that the physician will lose a lawsuit based on negligence.

Further reading

Accreditation Association for Ambulatory Health Care 2000 Accreditation handbook for ambulatory healthcare. Accreditation Association for Ambulatory Health Care, Wilmette, IL

Adamic M, Troilius A, Adatto M, et al 2007 Vascular lasers and IPLS: guidelines for care from the European Society for Laser Dermatology (ESLD). Journal of Cosmetic and Laser Therapy 9(2):113-124

Alam M, et al 2003 A prospective trial of fungal colonization after laser resurfacing of the face: correlation between culture positivity and symptoms of pruritus. Dermatologic Surgery 29(3):255-260

Alster TS, Lupton JR 2002 Prevention and treatment of side effects and complications of cutaneous laser resurfacing. Plastic and Reconstructive Surgery 109(1):308-316; discussion 317-318

Anvari B, et al 1998 A comparative study of human skin thermal response to sapphire contact and cryogen spray cooling. IEEE Transactions Biomedical Engineering 45(7):934-941

Ashinoff R, Levine VJ, Soter NA 1995 Allergic reactions to tattoo pigment after laser treatment. Dermatologic Surgery 21(4): 291-294

Avram MM, et al 2009 Hypertrophic scarring of the neck following ablative fractional carbon dioxide laser resurfacing. Lasers in Surgery and Medicine 41(3):185-188

Babilas P, et al 2010 Intense pulsed light (IPL): a review. Lasers in Surgery and Medicine 42(2):93-104

Badawi A, et al 2011 Retrospective analysis of non-ablative scar treatment in dark skin types using the sub-millisecond Nd:YAG 1,064 nm laser. Lasers in Surgery and Medicine 43(2):130-136

Bernstein EF 2006 Laser treatment of tattoos. Clinical Dermatology 24(1):43-55

Bernstein LJ, et al 1997 The short- and long-term side effects of carbon dioxide laser resurfacing. Dermatologic Surgery 23(7):519-525

Bolognia JL, Jorizzo JL, Rapini RP 2008 Dermatology, vol 2. 2nd edn. Mosby Elsevier, Philadelphia

Breadon JY, Barnes CA 2007 Comparison of adverse events of laser and light-assisted hair removal systems in skin types IV-VI. Journal of Drugs in Dermatology 6(1):40-46

Campbell TM, Goldman MP 2010 Adverse events of fractionated carbon dioxide laser: review of 373 treatments. Dermatologic Surgery 36(11):1645-1650

Casey AS, Goldberg D 2008 Guidelines for laser hair removal. Journal of Cosmetic and Laser Therapy 10(1):24-33

Chan HH, et al 2002 Clinical application of lasers in Asians. Dermatologic Surgery 28(7):556-563

Chan NP, et al 2010 The use of non-ablative fractional resurfacing in Asian acne scar patients. Lasers in Surgery and Medicine 42(10):710-715

Choudhary S, et al 2010 Lasers for tattoo removal: a review. Lasers in Medical Science 25(5):619-627

Chowdhury MM, Harris S, Lanigan SW 2001 Potassium titanyl phosphate laser treatment of resistant port-wine stains. British Journal of Dermatology 144(4):814-817

Clark C, et al 2004 Treatment of superficial cutaneous vascular lesions: experience with the KTP 532 nm laser. Lasers in Medical Science 19(1):1-5

Drosner M, Adatto M 2005 Photo-epilation: guidelines for care from the European Society for Laser Dermatology (ESLD). Journal of Cosmetic and Laser Therapy 7(1):33-38

England RW, Vogel P, Hagan L 2002 Immediate cutaneous hypersensitivity after treatment of tattoo with Nd:YAG laser: a case report and review of the literature. Annals of Allergy, Asthma and Immunology 89(2):215-217

Fitzpatrick RE, Goldman MP 1994 Tattoo removal using the alexandrite laser. Archives of Dermatology 130(12):1508-1514

Fitzpatrick RE, Lupton JR 2000 Successful treatment of treatment-resistant laser-induced pigment darkening of a cosmetic tattoo. Lasers in Surgery and Medicine 27(4):358-361

Furrow BF, Greaney TL, Johnson SH, Jost TS, et al 1997 Liability in health care law, 3rd edn. West Publishing, St Paul, MN

Goh CL 2003 Comparative study on a single treatment response to long pulse Nd:YAG lasers and intense pulse light therapy for hair removal on skin type IV to VI – is longer wavelengths lasers preferred over shorter wavelengths lights for assisted hair removal. Journal of Dermatologic Treatment 14(4):243-247

Goldberg DJ 2007 Laser dermatology: pearls and problems. Blackwell, Oxford, p ix, 188

Graber EM, Tanzi EL, Alster TS 2008 Side effects and complications of fractional laser photothermolysis: experience with 961 treatments. Dermatologic Surgery 34(3):301-305; discussion 305-307

Grevelink JM, et al 1996 Laser treatment of tattoos in darkly pigmented patients: efficacy and side effects. Journal of the American Academy of Dermatology 34(4):653-656

Grimes PE, et al 2001 Laser resurfacing-induced hypopigmentation: histologic alterations and repigmentation with topical photochemotherapy. Dermatologic Surgery 27(6):515-520

Gundogan C, et al 2004 [Repigmentation of persistent laser-induced hypopigmentation after tattoo ablation with the excimer laser]. Hautarzt 55(6):549-552

Hardaway CA, Ross EV, Paithankar DY 2002 Non-ablative cutaneous remodeling with a 1.45 microm mid-infrared diode laser: phase II. Journal of Cosmetic and Laser Therapy 4(1):9-14

Ho WS, et al 2004 Treatment of port wine stains with intense pulsed light: a prospective study. Dermatologic Surgery 30(6):887-890; discussion 890-891

Ho WS, et al 2006 Use of onion extract, heparin, allantoin gel in prevention of scarring in Chinese patients having laser removal of tattoos: a prospective randomized controlled trial. Dermatologic Surgery 32(7):891-896

Hunzeker CM, Weiss ET, Geronemus RG 2009 Fractionated CO_2 laser resurfacing: our experience with more than 2000 treatments. Aesthetic Surgery Journal 29(4):317-322

Iyer S, Fitzpatrick RE 2005 Long-pulsed dye laser treatment for facial telangiectasias and erythema: evaluation of a single purpuric pass versus multiple subpurpuric passes. Dermatologic Surgery 31(8 pt 1):898-903

Izikson L, Avram M, Anderson RR 2008 Transient immunoreactivity after laser tattoo removal: Report of two cases. Lasers in Surgery and Medicine 40(4):231-232

Joint Commission International 2005 Joint Commission International accreditation standards for ambulatory care, 2005. Joint Commission International, Oakbrook Terrace, IL, p v

Kauvar ANB, Hruza GJ 2005 Principles and practices in cutaneous laser surgery. Taylor & Francis, Boca Raton, p 815

Kelly KM, et al 1999 Cryogen spray cooling in combination with nonablative laser treatment of facial rhytides. Archives of Dermatology 135(6):691-694

Khan R 2001 Lasers in plastic surgery. Journal of Tissue Viability 11(3):103-107, 110-112

Kono T, et al 2006 Comparison study of a traditional pulsed dye laser versus a long-pulsed dye laser in the treatment of early childhood hemangiomas. Lasers in Surgery and Medicine 38(2):112-115

Kuperman-Beade M, Levine VJ, Ashinoff R 2001 Laser removal of tattoos. American Journal of Clinical Dermatology 2(1): 21-25

Lapidoth M, Aharonowitz G 2004 Tattoo removal among Ethiopian Jews in Israel: tradition faces technology. Journal of the American Academy of Dermatology 51(6):906-909

Laubach HJ, et al 2006 Skin responses to fractional photothermolysis. Lasers in Surgery and Medicine 38(2):142-149

Levine VJ, Geronemus RG 1995 Adverse effects associated with the 577- and 585-nanometer pulsed dye laser in the treatment of cutaneous vascular lesions: a study of 500 patients. Journal of the American Academy of Dermatology 32(4):613-617

Mahmoud BH, et al 2010 Safety and efficacy of erbium-doped yttrium aluminum garnet fractionated laser for treatment of acne scars in type IV to VI skin. Dermatologic Surgery 36(5):602-609

Manuskiatti W, Fitzpatrick RE, Goldman MP 1999 Long-term effectiveness and side effects of carbon dioxide laser resurfacing for photoaged facial skin. Journal of the American Academy of Dermatology 40(3):401-411

Moreno-Arias GA, Castelo-Branco C, Ferrando J 2002 Side-effects after IPL photodepilation. Dermatologic Surgery 28(12): 1131-1134

Nanni CA, Alster TS 1998 Complications of carbon dioxide laser resurfacing. An evaluation of 500 patients. Dermatologic Surgery 24(3):315-320

Neaman KC, et al 2010 Outcomes of fractional CO_2 laser application in aesthetic surgery: a retrospective review. Aesthetic Surgery Journal 30(6):845-852

Nelson AA, Lask GP 2011 Principles and practice of cutaneous laser and light therapy. Clinical Plastic Surgery 38(3): 427-436

Nelson JS, et al 1995 Dynamic epidermal cooling during pulsed laser treatment of port-wine stain. A new methodology with preliminary clinical evaluation. Archives of Dermatology 131(6):695-700

Nelson JS, et al 1996 Dynamic epidermal cooling in conjunction with laser-induced photothermolysis of port wine stain blood vessels. Lasers in Surgery and Medicine 19(2):224-229

Olbricht SM, et al 1987 Complications of cutaneous laser surgery. A survey. Archives of Dermatology 123(3):345-349

Prado A, et al 2008 Full-face carbon dioxide laser resurfacing: a 10-year follow-up descriptive study. Plastic and Reconstructive Surgery 121(3):983-993

Rao J, Golden TA, Fitzpatrick RE 2002 Atypical mycobacterial infection following blepharoplasty and full-face skin resurfacing with CO_2 laser. Dermatologic Surgery 28(8):768-771; discussion 771

Radmanesh M, et al 2002 Leukotrichia developed following application of intense pulsed light for hair removal. Dermatologic Surgery 28(7):572-574; discussion 574

Radmanesh M, et al 2008 Burning, paradoxical hypertrichosis, leukotrichia and folliculitis are four major complications of intense pulsed light hair removal therapy. Journal of Dermatologic Treatment 19(6):360-363

Radmanesh M 2009 Paradoxical hypertrichosis and terminal hair change after intense pulsed light hair removal therapy. Journal of Dermatologic Treatment 20(1):52-54

Raulin C, et al 1999 Treatment of port-wine stains with a noncoherent pulsed light source: a retrospective study. Archives of Dermatology 135(6):679-683

Raulin C, et al 2004 [Excimer laser. Treatment of iatrogenic hypopigmentation following skin resurfacing]. Hautarzt 55(8):746-748

Rheingold LM, Fater MC, Courtiss EH 1997 Compartment syndrome of the upper extremity following cutaneous laser surgery. Plastic and Reconstructive Surgery 99(5):1418-1420

Sriprachya-anunt S, et al 2002 Facial resurfacing in patients with Fitzpatrick skin type IV. Lasers in Surgery and Medicine 30(2):86-92

Tanzi EL, Williams CM, Alster TS 2003 Treatment of facial rhytides with a nonablative 1,450-nm diode laser: a controlled clinical and histologic study. Dermatologic Surgery 29(2):124-128

Torezan LA, Osorio N, Neto CF 2000 Development of multiple warts after skin resurfacing with CO_2 laser. Dermatologic Surgery 26(1):70-72

Trelles MA 2004 Laser resurfacing today and the 'cook book' approach: a recipe for disaster? Journal of Cosmetic Dermatology 3(4):237-241

Vlachos SP, Kontoes PP 2002 Development of terminal hair following skin lesion treatments with an intense pulsed light source. Aesthetic Plastic Surgery 26(4):303-307

Ward PD, Baker SR 2008 Long-term results of carbon dioxide laser resurfacing of the face. Archives of Facial Plastic Surgery 10(4):238-243; discussion 244-245

Wareham WJ, et al 2009 Adverse effects reported in pulsed dye laser treatment for port wine stains. Lasers in Medical Science 24(2):241-246

Page numbers followed by 'f' indicate figures, 't' indicate tables, and 'b' indicate boxes.